GERIATRIC DEPRESSION

ALSO FROM GARY J. KENNEDY

Geriatric Mental Health Care:
A Treatment Guide for Health Professionals

Geriatric Depression
A Clinical Guide

GARY J. KENNEDY

THE GUILFORD PRESS
New York   London

© 2015 The Guilford Press
A Division of Guilford Publications, Inc.
370 Seventh Avenue, Suite 1200, New York, NY 10001
www.guilford.com

Printed in the United States of America

This book is printed on acid-free paper.

Last digit is print number: 9   8   7   6   5   4   3   2   1

The author has checked with sources believed to be reliable in his efforts to
provide information that is complete and generally in accord with the standards
of practice that are accepted at the time of publication. However, in view of the
possibility of human error or changes in behavioral, mental health, or medical
sciences, neither the author, nor the editors and publisher, nor any other party
who has been involved in the preparation or publication of this work warrants
that the information contained herein is in every respect accurate or complete,
and they are not responsible for any errors or omissions or the results obtained
from the use of such information. Readers are encouraged to confirm the
information contained in this book with other sources.

Library of Congress Cataloging-in-Publication Data
Kennedy, Gary J., 1948– , author.
  Geriatric depression : a clinical guide / by Gary J. Kennedy.
    p. ; cm.
  Includes bibliographical references and index.
  ISBN 978-1-4625-1986-6 (hardcover : alk. paper)
  I. Title.
  [DNLM: 1. Depressive Disorder—therapy.   2. Aged—psychology.
WM 171.5]
  RC537.5
  618.97′68527—dc23

                                                    2015000366

To my wife, Jenny—
my first and favorite editor

About the Author

Gary J. Kennedy, MD, is Director of the Division of Geriatric Psychiatry and of the Fellowship Training Program at Montefiore Medical Center and Professor of Psychiatry and Behavioral Sciences at Albert Einstein College of Medicine, Bronx, New York. Dr. Kennedy is board certified in Geriatric Psychiatry and Psychosomatic Medicine. He is a past president of the American Association for Geriatric Psychiatry and a past chair of the Geriatric Mental Health Foundation. Dr. Kennedy is a recipient of an Award for Excellence in Program Innovation from the Archstone Foundation, an Exemplary Psychiatrist Award from the National Alliance for Mental Illness, and the 2014 Julia and Leo Forchheimer Foundation Lifetime Achievement Award. His research has focused on suicidal ideation, the epidemiology of depression and dementia, psychiatric services in primary care, and novel approaches to building bridges between community-based agencies and academic medical centers. His book *Geriatric Mental Health Care: A Treatment Guide for Health Professionals* received a Book of the Year Award in Gerontology from the *American Journal of Nursing* and in 2014 was listed as one of 100 Great Books for the Social Worker's Library by MSWOnlinePrograms.

Preface

Depression in late life is a paradox. The overwhelming majority of older persons are not depressed, yet advanced age and depressed mood are often thought of as cause and effect. Depression is most often a transient emotion, but it can be a crippling illness. As an illness it is eminently treatable, yet difficult to bring to full recovery. Persistent depressive illnesses are a major cause of suffering and disability, yet resources to address the personal and social impact of depression do not approximate the magnitude of need. Depression and physical disability go hand in hand, one causing the other in reciprocal fashion. Depression is associated with structural brain changes and cognitive dysfunction. Given the anatomy of depression, it is not surprising that use of anti-depressant prescriptions has increased severalfold among both younger and older adults. However, more treatment has not resulted in better treatment. Strategies to maximize recovery are well characterized but rarely employed. Despite exciting advances in our understanding of neural circuitry, the aging brain, and cognitive and interpersonal processes, therapeutic advances seem more incremental than dramatic. Although a breakthrough in the treatment of Alzheimer's disease is eagerly expected, none is anticipated for late-life depression.

And yet, the current portrait of depression among older adults need not cause pessimism. Rather, the very complexity of depression in late life implies an array of possible interventions, provided we get beyond the prejudice that aging is an illness better left alone.

The phenomenon of the compression of morbidity into the last years of life adds urgency to the argument for expanding access to evidence-based interventions for depression. Compression of morbidity refers to the increase in the active lifespan, that period when the older individual can enjoy relative independence, which for 30 years has outstripped the increase in total lifespan. As a result, disability and dependency are being compressed into the final years of life. This means that although the number of older persons with significant morbidity will increase as the older population grows, the proportion of older adults who are disabled will decline. This development, first described in the 1980s by Fries (Fries, Bruce, & Chakravarty, 2011) and subsequently confirmed by Cutler, Ghosh, and Landrum (2013), has grown despite the increasing prevalence of dementia, but it cannot be sustained unless the gains in independence late in life continue to outpace the gains in life expectancy. As a result, the public health imperative for a more aggressive stance toward depression is obvious.

This book grew out of my decades of teaching, training, research, and personal practice as a geriatric psychiatrist. It aspires to balance the scientific evidence regarding depression that students and trainees require with the pragmatism that practitioners demand. The initial chapter examines the epidemiology and terminology of depression both in scientific and common usage, as well as that described in DSM-5 (American Psychiatric Association, 2013). Although the focus is on persons 65 and older, the coverage on interventions and depression in the context of physical illness is relevant to a far larger population. Competence in treating depression in older individuals facilitates the care of younger people, particularly those with comorbid physical conditions. This book also offers insights into how depression care can be integrated—coordinated across diverse service settings from office-based practices of mental health providers to primary care, home care agencies, and nursing homes. Indeed, the burden of interventions for depressed persons is now and will increasingly be carried by professionals other than those in mental health. Hence the need for a source that provides guidance to the broadest audience of health professionals, including mental health practitioners.

Of course, not every reader will read every page. I have included numerous tables to guide readers with varying levels of interest and experience. Topics not typically seen in depression care texts—including etiology, diet, exercise, and prevention—are covered precisely because their absence would leave a void in both the practitioners' needs and the public's expectations. Healthy older adults want to stay healthy, and they expect providers to know more than "pills and talk" therapy. Chapters on the psychotherapies, other psychosocial interventions, and suicide are not meant to make readers experts in the field. Rather, they describe elements from the simple to the complex that can be incorporated into standard practice or require referral to a specialist. Similarly, the chapter on electroconvulsive therapy prepares the reader to discuss the treatment with patients and their families, whose fear and skepticism will most often pose a barrier. The ultimate goal is to give the reader a diverse set of resources to help adults overcome depression. The practitioner who is an optimistic, knowledgeable companion during the course of treatment is surely the best antidote to depression.

Acknowledgments

First, I thank the patients, families, and health care providers who have shared their sorrows and satisfactions with me and have motivated my writing. To the students, trainees, and fellows I have worked with, their success is a gratifying reminder that one teaches in order to learn. Thanks to the Leslie and Roslyn Goldstein Foundation for support that made it possible to devote time to this project. Support from the United Jewish Appeal–Federation of New York and the New York Foundation for Eldercare gave me access to systems of care that are critical to the well-being of older adults and their families but too often are absent from medical education. I thank the American Association for Geriatric Psychiatry, which champions the mental health of older Americans. Regarding colleagues and mentors, I thank Byram Karasu, the Chairman and Silverman Professor of Psychiatry and Behavioral Science at the Albert Einstein College of Medicine; Donna Cohen and Carl Eisdorfer, whose enthusiasm for geriatrics spurred my ambition; David Hamerman and Nancy Dubler, whose humanism continues to inspire just as it did during my first days at Montefiore; the leadership, staff, and residents of the Margaret Tietz Center for Nursing Care and Rehabilitation, who have taught me the meaning of quality in long-term care; faculty members Alessandra Scalmati and Mirnova Ceïde of the Division of Geriatric Psychiatry at Montefiore, whose zeal for teaching is remarkable; and Laurie Jacobs and all my colleagues in the Division of Geriatric Medicine and the physicians, nurses, and social workers whose work I so admire. Finally, I thank the editorial team at The Guilford Press, whose faith and patience brought this work to print.

Contents

CHAPTER 1

The Problem of Depression in Late Life

Depressive disorders are emerging as a leading cause of disability for older adults, soon to be second only to heart disease (Chapman & Perry, 2008). Depression is the third leading contributor to the global disease burden, surpassing the psychotic disorders and dementia (Collins et al., 2011). By 2030, major depressive disorder is expected to be second leading cause of disability worldwide after HIV and AIDS and the number one cause of disability in the developed nations (Mathers & Loncar, 2006; Mitchell, Vaze, & Rau, 2009). As a result, the public heath imperative to reduce late-life disability and to compress morbidity into the very end of the lifespan is immense. As mentioned in the introduction, the proportion of older adults who are disabled is declining at the same time that the absolute number of seniors is increasing. Improved treatment of depression will play a major role in furthering this phenomenon. At the same time, depressed older persons are less likely than younger persons to recognize depression symptoms as an illness (Alexopoulos et al., 2004) and less likely to present depression as an initial complaint to their primary care physicians, who treat depressed persons far more often than mental health specialists. Awareness of the situations and conditions associated with the emergence of depression is critical to treatment.

The first part of this chapter examines the epidemiology of depression in late life, offering a picture of who is most likely to be depressed and the extent of the problem. The second discusses diagnosis and presents an overview of the many forms that depression can take in older people.

EPIDEMIOLOGY OF DEPRESSION

The incidence and prevalence of depression vary widely among older adults based on how the condition is defined, where it is assessed, and the generation under observation. Although the loss of friends and family is an inevitable consequence of aging, it is declining health and the onset of disability that are the twin determinants of the majority of depressive symptoms and disorders in late life. Indeed, as discussed below, depression is rare among healthy older community residents. Yet as the absolute number of older Americans increases, the number of those with poor health and dependency will also increase.

Incidence

Incidence is the number of individuals developing a condition within a specific period of observation. Incidence rate appears with a time frame, the number of new cases divided by the period of observation denoted as person-years. In the community-based Cache County survey using multiple assessment methods, from 1 to 2.5% of adults ages 65–100 developed a first episode of depression over the course of 1 year. Face-to-face interviews demonstrated incidence rates for any type of depressive disorder of 1.3/100 person-years for men and 1.9 for women. When evidence that an antidepressant had been prescribed was included, rates grew to 1.5 for men and 2.3 for women. Adding information from postmortem interviews with collateral informants yielded rates of 2.1 for men and 2.6 for women. Of those with no prior history, the rates for major depression fell to 0.78 for men and 0.87 for women. Rates for minor depression were 1.9 for men and 2.4 for women. Advanced age did not predict incidence (Norton, Skoog, Toone, et al., 2006).

In a systematic review that focused on persons ages 70 and older, Büchtemann et al. (2012) examined 20 studies of depression incidence and associated characteristics. In 14 studies, incidence was defined by categorical criteria obtained from structured interviews with diagnostic instruments. In the remaining 6, incidence was defined by the more easily obtained dimensional criteria of a clinically significant symptom score. Categorical diagnostic measures identify persons in need of treatment. Dimensional diagnostic measures more accurately identify those at risk and as such denote "probable" depression. However Büchtemann et al. (2012) found the incidence of major depression not to be higher among persons ages 70 and older than among young and middle aged adults. Beyond age 70 neither female gender nor advancing age was consistently or substantially associated with major depression. Rather, physical morbidity, disability, and psychosocial events such as personal losses, change in residence, and diminished autonomy overwhelmed the contribution of age and gender as defining elements of risk. Although the onset of major depression in old age was rare, elevations in depressive symptoms were not. The incidence rate of major depression ranged from 0.2–14.1/100 person-years. The incidence of clinically significant depressive symptoms was 6.8/100 person-years.

Prevalence

Prevalence estimates are snapshots depicting how widespread an illness or condition is at one point in time. As such they are far more common than incidence data, which requires the assembly of a healthy cohort and subsequent observation to determine who remains well and who becomes sick. Prevalence can be used to identify associated characteristics but is less informative about etiology, and risk factors for onset and persistence of illness. Although acknowledging the lack of definitive prevalence estimates, the Committee on the Mental Health Workforce for Geriatric Populations of the Institute of Medicine (Eden et al., 2012) concluded that from 5.6 million to 8 million older Americans have one or more mental health or substance use conditions. Depressive disorders and dementia-related behavioral and psychiatric symptoms were the most prevalent. This means from 14 to 20% of older Americans are affected.

Focused only on noninstitutionalized adults 65 years of age and older, the Health Retirement Study found an age-related increase in depressive symptoms as measured by the Center for Epidemiologic Studies Depression Scale. Ten percent of men ages 65–69 were depressed, compared to 15% of women. But by age 85 the prevalence increased to 18% among both men and women (Federal Interagency Forum on Aging-Related Statistics, 2012). But methods using more exacting standards yield different results.

As reported in the Weekly Morbidity and Mortality Review (Centers for Disease Control and Prevention, 2010) the Centers for Disease Control and Prevention (CDC) analyzed Behavioral Risk Factor Surveillance System (BRFSS) survey data from 2006 and 2008 to determine the prevalence of current depression among 235,067 adults in 45 states, the District of Columbia, Puerto Rico, and the U.S. Virgin Islands. Current depression was defined as meeting BRFSS criteria for either "major" or "other" depression. Criteria were based on respondent answers to the eight-item Patient Health Questionnaire (PHQ-8). The questionnaire, usually with nine items, is commonly used in primary care settings to screen and diagnose depressive disorders. The nine-item Patient Health Questionnaire (PHQ-9) is discussed in more detail later in this chapter and can be seen in Figure 1.1. The CDC study omitted question 9 from the PHQ, which queries thoughts of death or self-harm. Interviewers did not have access to clinical risk assessors for suicide and could not ethically inquire about risk without access to a potential intervention. Respondents answering yes to either the depressed mood or anhedonia question plus four others lasting "more than half of the days" during the previous 2 weeks met criteria for major depression. Those responding yes to either depressed mood or anhedonia and at least one other item met criteria for "other depression," which might include dysthymia, minor or subsyndromal depression. Of those ages 65 and older, 1.6% (95% confidence interval [CI] 1.4–1.8) met criteria for major depression, and 5.2% (95% CI 4.9–5.6) for other depression. The combined percentage of 6.8 as well as the figures for major and other depression were lower among those 65 and older than for any other age group. Including all ages, 9.0% met criteria for current depression, including 3.4% for major depression. The prevalence of major depression increased from 2.8% in young adulthood (ages 18–24 years) to 4.6% in middle age (45–64 years), but declined among those ages 65 and older.

Similarly, data from the National Comorbidity Survey Replication (Byers et al., 2010) demonstrated a statistically reliable decline in rates of both depression and anxiety disorders with advancing age. The prevalence of depression was higher among women. However, anxiety disorders were more common than depression across all age groups, for men and women. These two studies are noteworthy for the similarity of

Two-question screening with the PHQ-2:

Over the last 2 weeks, how often have you been bothered by the following problems?	Not at all	Several days	More than half the days	Nearly every day
A. Little interest or pleasure in doing things?	0	1	2	3
B. Feeling down, depressed, or hopeless?	0	1	2	3

If A + B is 3 or greater, ask the following:

Over the last 2 weeks, how often have you been bothered by the following problems?	Not at all	Several days	More than half the days	Nearly every day
Feeling tired or having little energy?	0	1	2	3
Poor appetite or overeating?	0	1	2	3
Trouble falling or staying asleep, or sleeping too much?	0	1	2	3
Feeling bad about yourself—or that you are a failure or have let yourself or your family down?	0	1	2	3
Trouble concentrating on things, such as reading the newspaper or watching television?	0	1	2	3
Moving or speaking so slowly that other people could have noticed? Or the opposite—being so fidgety or restless that you have been moving around a lot more than usual?	0	1	2	3
Thoughts that you would be better off dead, or of hurting yourself?	0	1	2	3

FIGURE 1.1. The nine-item Patient Health Questionnaire (PHQ-9): Screening questions and complete assessment. Copyright originally held by Pfizer, Inc. Duplication approved for clinical use. Now designated as in the public domain. Retrieved June 30, 2014, from *www.phqscreeners.com*.

findings despite the use of different sampling procedures and diagnostic methodologies. But both offer a conservative, perhaps overly conservative, view of depression among older adults for a number of reasons (Byers et al., 2010). Lowered prevalence may reflect selective mortality in which vulnerable depressed individuals die before reaching older age. Other conditions associated with depression may result in change from community to institutional residence, making the older adult inaccessible for survey studies. Indeed, the prevalence of clinically relevant depressive symptoms increases to one senior in four in primary care, assisted living, and acute-care settings (Alexopoulos et al., 2005b). Frailty, cognitive impairment, and sensory deficits may make participation difficult or unreliable. Older adults may be less comfortable expressing depressive symptoms or experience their distress more in terms of anxiety than mood disturbance. Apathy, irritability, and social withdrawal may be more characteristic of late-life depression. Depressive symptoms associated with a physical condition or ascribed to bereavement may not be attributed to mental illness, yet amplify disability and distress in a clinically significant fashion (Pickett et al., 2014a). Efforts to distinguish primary from secondary depression among older adults do not effectively direct interventions.

Among community-residing older adults, declining health and increasing disability are the major predictors of both the emergence and persistence of clinically significant depressive symptoms (Kennedy et al., 1990, 1991). As a result, the prevalence of all forms of depression would be expected to be higher in primary care settings given the association of physical illness and disability with depressive symptoms. At least 6% of older primary care patients meet criteria for major depression (O'Connor et al., 2009), with another 6% meeting criteria for minor depression or dysthymia. An additional 10% meet criteria for subsyndromal depression, meaning they score above the recovery threshold of the Hamilton Depression Rating Scale (HAM-D) and may be at risk for a major depressive episode (Lyness et al., 1999).

In sum, the incidence of major depression is low among community-dwelling older adults. However, the prevalence of clinically significant depressive symptoms and disorders among primary care patients is substantial. An examination of age per se suggests an optimistic view toward depression in late life. Rather than age, it is the age-related experience of illness, disability, and loss that determine much of the risk of old-age affective disorders. And because each of these is a relatively discrete event, detection and interventions are feasible. The rest of this chapter focuses on detection and examines the varying ways that depression can present.

Diagnosing Depression in Late Life

Diagnosing depression as an illness is a challenge in older adults. Criteria for a major depressive disorder include five symptoms, one of which must be either depressed mood or loss of interest in pleasurable activities nearly every day for the previous 2 weeks (DSM-5; American Psychiatric Association, 2013). However, the emotional disturbance of major depressive disorder may not be the most disabling aspect of the illness. If there is loss of interest compounded by disturbances in physical and cognitive function an episode of major depression may be present. As a result one need not have depressed mood to have a major depressive disorder. Supporting symptoms include change in appetite, insomnia or hypersomnia, psychomotor agitation or retardation, fatigue, feelings of worthlessness or excess guilt, difficulty concentrating, and recurrent thoughts of death, dying, or suicide. All must directly cause significant distress or social impairment. The disability the patient experiences must not be due to drugs, medications, or medical conditions, and symptoms must not simply be the effects of bereavement. A major depressive disorder may be diagnosed during a period of bereavement if the distress exceeds expectations based on the individual's history, cultural norms, and clinical judgment. These criteria encompass many different forms of depression, including recurrent or treatment-resistant depression, depression with psychosis, and depression with anxiety, each of which may require differing forms of medication and psychotherapy. Among younger persons depressive disorders most commonly occur exclusive of concurrent physical illness. However, concurrent physical illness is the norm rather than the exception among older patients. The question the practitioner must ask is "Is there some form of a depressive disorder that might be adding excess, potentially reversible disability to the patient's condition?"

The PHQ-9 is commonly used in primary care settings to assist in the screening and diagnosis of major depressive disorders. (The first two questions alone, the PHQ-2, can also be used as a screening instrument.) At a score of 10 or greater, the nine depression items achieve a sensitivity of 88% and specificity of 88% for major depressive disorder among primary care patients, as compared to a structured diagnostic interview from a mental health professional (Kroenke & Spitzer, 2002). As shown in Figure 1.1, the PHQ-9 questions closely resemble the DSM-5 array of depressive symptoms and similarly require either depressed mood or loss of interest and pleasure to be present most days in the previous 2 weeks. The PHQ-9 score can be used as a severity indicator for the initiation or modification of treatment, as well as for justifying the request for psychiatric consultation (see Table 1.1). As shown in Table 1.2, the serial administration of the PHQ-9 can be used to assess treatment response and the adequacy of antidepressant treatment (Oxman, 2003). As discussed in Chapter 2, executive dysfunction is a predictor of poor response to treatment for depression. Brief assessments of executive dysfunction can be found in Chapter 2 and in Table 2.2.

Assessing Suicide Risk

As discussed in more detail in Chapter 9, older adults represented 13% of the U.S. population in 2010 but accounted for 15% of suicides (Murphy, Xu, & Kochanek, 2013). As noted above, the ninth item of the PHQ-9 is an initial screen for suicidal ideation and should not be omitted. When patients express thoughts of death or suicide or have several risk factors (even if denying thoughts of death), the level of suicide risk should be assessed. Table 1.3 outlines procedural guidelines for the practitioner. When risk is not high, consider referral for cognitive-behavioral therapy (CBT) for suicidality, described in Chapter 4.

TABLE 1.1. Indications for the Initiation of Antidepressant Treatment Based on the PHQ-9

PHQ-9 score	Depression severity	Clinician response
1–4	None	None
5–9	Mild to moderate	If not currently treated, rescreen in 2 weeks. If currently treated, optimize antidepressant and rescreen in 2 weeks.
10–15	Major depressive disorder	Initiate antidepressant.
15 and above	Major depressive disorder	Initiate antidepressant, obtain psychiatric consultation if suicidality or psychosis suspected.

TABLE 1.2. Prescriber Response Guidelines at 4 Weeks Based on the PHQ-9 and the Sequenced Treatment Alternatives to Relieve Depression (STAR*D) Studies

PHQ-9 score or change	Outcome	Clinician response
No decrease or increase	Nonresponse	Switch medication.
Decrease of 2–4 points	Partial response	Add medication.
Decrease 5 or more points	Response	Maintain medication.
PHQ-9 < 5	Remission	Maintain medication.

TABLE 1.3. Practitioner-Based Interventions to Reduce the Risk of Late-Life Suicide

If few risk factors are present:
- Screen annually for depression.
- Advanced directives (Patient Self-Determination Act).
- Encourage abstinence or moderation in alcohol intake.
- Encourage smoking cessation.
- Encourage social engagement.

If several risks factors are present but suicidal ideas are denied:
- As above if indicated, and . . .
  o Optimize treatment of depression, anxiety, insomnia, pain, alcohol abuse.

If thoughts of suicide are present but without intent or a plan:
- As above if indicated, and . . .
  o Make family aware of elevated risk and ensure practitioner availability.
  o Instruct family or third party to remove lethal means and alcohol.
  o Identify reasons to live (concern for family, religion, life event goals).
  o Fix an appointment (not as needed); ask that family attend.

If lethal means are available, a plan is expressed, or intent is evident:
- Refer for emergency psychiatric evaluation (involuntary, if needed).
- Consider hospitalization, electroconvulsive therapy.

If suicide has been attempted, or countervailing forces are not available to prevent recurrent attempts:
- Refer for emergency psychiatric evaluation (involuntary, if needed).
- Hospitalize if intent not convincingly recanted or attempt is a recurrence.

Note. Adapted from Kennedy (2000, p. 237). Copyright 2000 by The Guilford Press. Adapted by permission.

Response, Remission, Relapse, and Recurrence

In studies of antidepressants or psychotherapy, the terms "response" and "remission" describe, respectively, patients who are made better and those who are made well by the intervention. "Partial response" describes patients who have improved but not to the extent of meeting criteria for a genuine response. The distinctions are important because of empirical findings regarding their association with prognosis both in the near and far term, and thereby the adequacy of therapy. The longer it takes a person to respond, the less likely he or she is to achieve remission and to subsequently recover. Chances of success are even lower if the response is only partial, which will predispose the person to relapse. Relapse is defined as an exacerbation of symptoms despite transient improvement. Similarly, meeting the more stringent criteria for remission means reducing the likelihood of recurrence. For clinical investigation the standard baseline measure of symptom severity is the Ham-D, with a score of 18–20, in addition to meeting DSM-5 criteria for major depression. Response is defined as a 50% reduction from the baseline in the total HAM-D score. Partial responses are defined as a reduction of 30% or more but less than 50%. For remission either a score of 10, or more stringently 7, must be reached. Stated differently, persons virtually free of depressive symptoms are least likely to have a subsequent episode of major depression, which is the definition of recurrent depression. An episode of major depression severe enough to require hospitalization or complicated by suicidal ideation is more likely to be followed by recurrence even when stringent criteria for remission attain.

In primary care settings, where the HAM-D may be less familiar, response and remission may be assessed though serial administrations of the PHQ-9 without having to calculate percentage change from baseline. As shown in Table 1.2, a 5-point decline indicates a response. Patients scoring 5 or less have achieved remission (Oxman, 2003). The score can be used as an objective measure, beyond the clinician's global impression of change, to discuss prognosis and the subsequent course of treatment. For the sake of convenience, the PHQ-9 may be administered by phone without sacrificing validity. Indeed, telephone administration may be less embarrassing (Allen, Cull, & Sharpe, 2003) and a more effective means of reducing mental health disparities among members of disadvantaged minority groups (Pickett et al., 2014b).

The balance of this chapter overviews the various ways in which depression can present in older people and their clinical implications.

DEPRESSIVE CONDITIONS
OTHER THAN MAJOR DEPRESSION

What follows is meant to help the reader navigate the scientific literature, which at times addresses the categorical entity of depressive disorders but also examines the dimensional conditions in which depressive symptoms are more or less present but do not reach the threshold of a disorder. Definitions of "subclinical," "subsyndromal," "minor," and "submajor" depression are confusing, with various investigators using DSM criteria and/or structured diagnostic interviews and symptom severity scores to characterize symptomatic individuals. DSM-5 describes three "other specified depressive disorders" that are not the aftermath of a major mood or psychotic disorder. Recurrent brief depression is defined by episodes that occur at least monthly with depressed mood plus four other criteria of a major disorder but do not last the requisite 2 weeks. Short-duration depressive episode contains the same symptom count but lasts from 4 to 13 days. Depressive episode with insufficient symptoms is defined by the presence of depressed mood, but with only one other criterion symptom of a major disorder, which lasts for 2 weeks. The utility of these designations for older adults and the providers who care for them remains to be determined.

In contrast, "minor depression," which appears in the appendix to DSM-IV (American Psychiatric Association, 1994), uses the same list of symptoms as major depression but requires only depressed mood plus one other symptom to meet criteria. Subsyndromal depression is generally used to distinguish persons whose number or duration of depressive symptoms does not conform to criteria for minor depression. Dysthymic disorder (persistent depressive disorder in DSM-5), defined as depressed mood plus one of eight other DSM criteria present most of the day more days than not over 2 or more years, is often included. However, each designation is associated with as much as a fivefold risk for the subsequent development of a major depressive episode (Lyness et al., 2007) as well as increased use of health services even without progression to a major disorder (Pickett et al., 2014a). These entities may be the prodrome for, or the residue of, a major depressive episode. They also represent a dimension of both symptom severity and duration. Nonetheless, a substantial number of patients in each category will experience a spontaneous remission of symptoms with no intervention. Self-assessed poor health, perceived lack of social support (Lyness et al., 2006), symptom severity, and general assessment of functioning (Lyness et al., 2009) may be the simplest, most reliable measures to predict the subsequent development of major depression. As a result, patients whose symptoms meet the definitions for these entities may be among the most logical population for interventions to prevent the onset and disability of major depressive disorders (see Chapter 9).

PSYCHOTIC DEPRESSION

Patients with psychotic depression, more appropriately described as delusional depression, have sustained irrational beliefs (delusions) in association with depressed mood. These delusions are often plausible. Psychotic depression should be suspected when the irrational belief focuses on somatic symptoms or around fears of a serious physical condition when there is no medical evidence to support the belief despite adequate examinations. Patients with somatic delusions visit multiple specialists and obtain repeated testing to identify problems that they "know" exist rather than for the purpose of seeking relief from persistent somatic "worries." The presence of delusions in association with major depression is not recognized in 25% of cases (Andreescu, Mulsant, & Peasley-Miklus, 2007). The careful assessment of depressed patients for the plausibility of their concerns would presumably reduce this rate.

Differential Diagnosis

Due to the obsessional yet plausible quality of the delusions, obsessive–compulsive disorder may seem a reasonable possibility. The difference between obsessive rumination and delusional thinking can be difficult to distinguish (DeBattista & Lembke, 2008). Body Dysmorphic disorder with psychosis, which is characterized by an irrational belief that one's physique is seriously flawed despite obvious evidence to the contrary, may also complicate the diagnostic consideration. Hypochondriasis is a common feature of delusional depression, misdirecting the diagnostician to a somatoform (somatic symptoms disorder in DSM-5) rather than a mood disorder. The distinction is important because body dysmorphic disorder responds to monotherapy with a selective serotonin reuptake inhibitor (SSRI; Phillips, 2004). Difficulty concentrating, deficits in executive function, and subjective complaints of impaired cognition suggestive of dementia are frequently seen. The occurrence of depression with hallucinations but not delusions in older adults suggests structural brain diseases, or bipolar or schizoaffective disorder. Other symptoms of a major depressive disorder may not be so prominent or severe, further distracting the practitioner from the correct diagnosis. Differentiating schizoaffective disorder from psychotic depression may also be difficult because of the inability to reliably differentiate the sequence of symptom emergence, and establish the presence of psychosis prior to depression (Rothschild et al., 2006).

BIPOLAR DEPRESSION

Occurring in approximately 0.5% of the U.S. population, type II bipolar disorder is characterized by recurrent major depressive episodes interspersed with periods of hypomania (Mitchell, Wilhelm, & Parker, 2001). Hypomania is defined as a disturbance in which mood is persistently and abnormally elevated, irritable, or expansive for at least 4 days' duration. Associated symptoms include grandiosity or inflated self-regard, decreased need for sleep, loquaciousness or pressured speech, flight of ideas, racing thoughts, distractibility, agitation, increased goal-directed activity, and pursuit of pleasures with high self-destructive potential. The symptoms represent an unequivocal, uncharacteristic, and socially disruptive change in behavior. The absence of psychosis and severe social impairment and the duration of symptoms for less than 1 week distinguish hypomania from the mania of type I bipolar disorder.

Because the social disruption may be minimal, and some of the symptoms may even seem beneficial, past episodes of hypomania may have been ignored or dismissed by the patient and family. Major depressive episodes also occur in type I bipolar disorder, in which the occurrence of one or more manic episodes is the distinguishing diagnostic feature. And there are mixed states in which criteria for both mania and major depression are present. As a result the term "bipolar depression" spans the spectrum of bipolar disorders. This broad, rather heterogeneous definition may explain why the array of proven treatments, especially for older patients, remains limited.

Among older adults with bipolar disorder, mania is a more frequent cause of hospitalization than depression (Sajatovic et al., 2005), but depression may account for more disability (Sachs et al., 2007). Worse, the results of present treatment for older adults with bipolar disorders are not remarkably better than those recorded prospectively from 1959 to 1985 (Angst & Presig, 1995). Indeed, few older persons with the disorder experience a full functional recovery despite symptom remission. Perlis et al. (2006a) prospectively assessed potential predictors of recurrent mood disturbance among 858 symptomatic patients ages 15 and older who subsequently recovered from an episode of bipolar illness. Of persons followed for up to 2 years, nearly half experienced a recurrence. And depressive episodes were twice as frequent as manic ones. The proportion of days depressed or anxious in the preceding year as well as residual symptoms of depression or mania at recovery predicted a subsequent depressive episode. Proportion of days with elevated mood in the preceding year, as well as residual symptoms of mania, were associated with a shorter time to the recurrence of a manic, mixed, or depressive episode. Impairments in cognitive speed and executive dysfunction (Gildengers et al., 2007; Murphy et al., 1999) and changes in subcortical brain structures are common (McDonald et al., 1991), further reducing the chances of return to full function.

Vascular Depression

Two groups, led by Krishnan (Krishnan, Doraiswamy, & Clary, 2001) and Alexopoulos (Alexopoulos et al., 1997), have described major depressive episodes occurring after age 55 associated with white matter changes on magnetic resonance images of the brain and executive dysfunction on measures of neuropsychological performance. White matter, in the center of the brain, allows communication to and from gray matter, the information-processing areas, and other parts of the body. As many as 50% of older adults experiencing a major depressive episode may have subcortical white matter changes (Krishnan et al., 2004). These patients are also more likely to have heart disease, hypertension, and diabetes. More important, executive dysfunction predicts delayed or absent response to antidepressant medication (Alexopoulos et al., 2008) and accelerates development of dementia (Alexopoulos et al., 2005b). Executive deficits may prevent the recovery of independence even when the mood disorder of a major depressive episode has fully remitted (Alexopoulos, Meyers, Young, et al., 2000).

Subsequently Alexopoulos and colleagues (2008) tested the hypothesis that depressed elders who fail to achieve remission have microstructural white matter abnormalities in cortico-striato-limbic networks. They used diffusion tensor imaging, a magnetic resonance imaging

(MRI) technique that displays the integrity of neural tracts connecting cortical and subcortical structures. This technique measures the extent to which water molecules in the brain exhibit diffuse (isotropic) versus directional (anisotropic) patterns of movement. The greater the diffusion tensor anisotropy, the greater the integrity and connectivity of the neural circuit or network. Lesser anisotropy is thought to represent disconnection between distributed cerebral networks. Among 23 older patients who had not achieved remission of depressive symptoms despite adequate dose and duration of antidepressant treatment, they found lower fractional anisotropy in multiple frontal limbic brain areas. The authors concluded that lower fractional anisotropy is associated with poor antidepressant response and may represent a neuroanatomical substrate that predisposes to geriatric depression.

However, the white matter changes and anisotropy associated with depression may convey other risks as well. In the Longitudinal Aging Study of Amsterdam, 2,965 adults with a mean age of 70 years and without a history of stroke were followed for 9 years or until the occurrence of a stroke. In participants with prior heart disease, but not in those without, clinically relevant depressive symptoms at baseline (hazard ratio [HR] 2.18; 95% CI 1.17–4.09) and the severity (range 0–60; HR 1.08; 95% CI 1.02–1.13) and chronicity (HR 3.51; 95% CI 1.13–10.93) of symptoms during follow-up were associated with stroke. The investigators concluded that symptoms of depression at baseline as well as their severity and persistence were associated with subsequent stroke (Wouts et al., 2008). I say more about white matter brain changes in the next chapter.

MIXED ANXIETY–DEPRESSION

Older adults may have clinically significant symptoms of both depression and anxiety, yet not meet formal criteria for either a depressive or anxiety disorder (unspecified depressive disorder in DSM-5). This syndrome of mixed anxiety and depression is associated with impaired social function, exacerbated disability due to physical illness, suicidality, and poor prognosis. The severity profile may shift back and forth from more anxious to more depressed, with one profile masking the presence of the other and making diagnosis difficult. For example, hallmark symptoms of anxiety disorders such as avoidance and realization that symptoms are out of the norm or "excessive" may not be readily apparent to the older person.

Avoidance rationales may seem reasonable on the surface, but upon examination are maladaptive. These include (1) excessive checking of financial records, medications, blood pressure, or the well-being of family members; (2) failure to accept assistive devices or home care services or to purchase needed items out of exaggerated concern for costs or loss of independence; (3) refusing to engage in socially supportive activities or family events out of fear of being perceived as "stupid" or "old" or burdensome; and (4) hoarding. Interestingly, fear of falling exists along with anxiety symptoms, but like the behaviors listed above does not seem excessive to the affected older adult. However, the word *excessive* may not conform to the older patient's perceptions. Asking "compared to others your age . . ." or "how much time do you spend worrying about . . ." may give a more telling picture of preoccupation and counterproductive consequences. Similarly, younger persons with phobias are more likely to acknowledge the irrationality of their fears. In contrast, "uncontrollability" distinguishes older but not younger patients who meet criteria for generalized anxiety disorder compared to those with subclinical anxiety. Clinic-based studies find little prevalence of anxiety disorders in the absence of comorbid depression (major depressive disorder with anxious distress in DSM-5) in contrast to community-based samples, in which discrete anxiety disorders do appear.

Further complicating the recognition of anxiety symptoms is their co-occurrence with medical conditions. Panic attacks due to angina or the hypoxemia of chronic obstructive pulmonary disease may be directly due to physiological processes yet still lead to agoraphobia. Corticosteroids and other medications can be anxiety provoking yet be accompanied by disability in excess of expectations. In summary, practitioners should be vigilant for symptoms of anxiety, not to stigmatize the genuine fears associated with the patient's physical condition or prognosis, but rather to detect the presence of a disorder whose diagnosis may justify intervention and promote autonomy. There are several antidepressant medications approved for the treatment of anxiety (see Table 3.1) that are preferred over benzodiazepines. Psychotherapies for depression and anxiety can be hybridized to address both (see Chapter 4 and Tables 4.1 and 4.2). Note that offering an intervention to an anxious person is bound to provoke anxiety. The presence of supportive family is invaluable not only to substantiate the diagnosis but also to assist with acceptance of the treatment (Mohlman et al., 2012).

AFFECTIVE SYNDROME OF ALZHEIMER'S DISEASE

Depressive symptoms are the most common neuropsychiatric manifestation of dementia. Depression is thought to be a risk factor for development of dementia, a symptom of dementia, and a separate diagnostic entity that can represent recurrence of a comorbid disorder (Kennedy & Kastenschmidt, 2010). As a result, efforts to characterize as well as treat depression in the dementias including Alzheimer's disease have been extensive. One expert group (Olin et al., 2002) described an affective syndrome of dementia captured by depressed mood, loss of positive affect, or loss of pleasure in activities plus two additional criteria, all lasting a minimum of 2 weeks. Additional symptoms included social isolation or withdrawal, disruption in sleep or appetite, psychomotor retardation, agitation, fatigue, loss of energy, irritability, feeling worthless, hopeless, or guilty, and morbid preoccupation (death, suicide).

However, in cross-sectional data from persons with dementia in the Cache County study (Lyketsos et al., 2001), apathy was the most common neuropsychiatric symptom, followed by depressed mood, agitation, aggression, and irritability. Depressed mood was more prevalent in vascular dementia. Hallucinations and delusions did not cluster with apathy, irritability, or depressed mood. The most common neuropsychiatric symptom profile was an affective syndrome characterized by apathy, depression, and irritability in more than a quarter of the sample. In another population-based study, motivation-related symptoms (disinterest, low energy, poor concentration) rather than mood disturbances were more prevalent. Notably there was no correlation between the presence of depressive symptoms and the patient's awareness of cognitive deficit (Berger et al., 1999). The Depression in Alzheimer's Disease Study (DIADS) enrolled patients meeting criteria for either a major depressive disorder or minor depression, or the less severe affective syndrome. Patients underwent a randomized, placebo-controlled trial of sertraline (Drye et al., 2011). Although participants on average achieved a 50% reduction in depressive symptoms, there was no statistically significant difference between sertraline and placebo. Nor was there a difference in outcomes based on major or minor depression status. But this is not to say that the depressive symptoms so prevalent in dementia are beyond intervention. Rather, behavioral management techniques taught to caregivers can have measureable and lasting benefits, as shown in chapter on psychotherapy. The hope offered caregivers by both the drug and placebo arms in DIADS may have had a genuine therapeutic effect that was not illusory.

CONCLUSION

Depression in late life may present as a disorder, a transient emotional state, or a symptom associated with a physical disorder or medication. The challenge is: What to do? The array of interventions, including reassurance and watchful waiting, follows in subsequent chapters. Table 1.4 briefly summarizes the forms of depression that practitioners may encounter. It is the presence of excess, potentially avoidable disability that compels intervention. More often than not, the promise of restoring function, and of preserving autonomy, is the determining factor in the patient's acceptance of treatment. For both the practitioner and the patient, it is a functional solution that is used to address the problematic definition of depression.

TABLE 1.4. Distinguishing Characteristics of Depressive Disorders and Syndromes

Disorder or syndrome	Criteria	Source
Major depressive disorder	Depressed mood or anhedonia, plus four other symptoms, almost every day for most of the day for at least 2 weeks, severe enough to cause a major change in personal function	DSM-5
Persistent depressive disorder (dysthymia in DSM-IV-TR)	Chronically depressed mood most days plus two additional symptoms, 2 years or more duration	DSM-5
Minor depression	Depressed mood plus one other symptom nearly every day for at least 2 weeks, severe enough to "represent a change from previous functioning"	DSM-IV
Subsyndromal, subclinical, submajor depression	No set definition; generally indicates the presence of depressive symptoms, but of insufficient duration, severity, or number to meet DSM-IV-TR criteria for major depressive disorder; often defined statistically on the basis of the diagnostic or symptom checklist instrument used in the study	Lyness et al. (2006)
Other specified depressive disorder	Recurrent brief depression; short-duration depressive episode; depressive episode with insufficient symptoms	DSM-5
Bipolar depression	Major depressive episodes in the context of prior episodes of hypomania (bipolar type II) or mania (bipolar type I)	DSM-5
Depression with anxious distress or with mixed features	Depressive disorder with significant symptoms of an anxiety disorder or bipolar I disorder in which mania and depression alternate over the period of a week	DSM-5
Depression due to other medical disorder	Major depressive episode caused by, rather than simply associated with, a physical illness (e.g., hypothyroidism) or treatment (e.g., interferon alpha)	DSM-5
Adjustment disorder with depressed mood	Disturbance in mood (depression, tearfulness, hopelessness) that follows within 3 months of a stressor and is excessively disruptive but self-limited to 6-month duration; not bereavement	DSM-5

(continued)

TABLE 1.4. *(continued)*

Disorder or syndrome	Criteria	Source
Complicated bereavement	Crippling grief that may meet criteria for major depressive disorder but includes (1) a sense of disbelief regarding the death, (2) anger, bitterness over the loss, (3) recurrent waves of painful yearning, (4) preoccupation with the loss, (5) intrusive thoughts related to the death, and (6) avoidance of situations and activities that remind the person of the loss	Shear et al. (2005)
Depression with psychotic features	Major depressive disorder accompanied by delusions, less often hallucinations; the delusional person may be preoccupied with somatic fears, guilt, or impoverishment	DSM-5
Affective syndrome of Alzheimer's disease	Depressed mood or "decreased positive affect or pleasure" (anhedonia) plus two additional symptoms of major depressive disorder; symptoms such as weight loss or social withdrawal should not simply be a manifestation of the dementia	Olin et al. (2002)
Late-onset depression	Major depressive episode with onset at age 55 or older	Alexopoulos et al. (1997)
Vascular depression	Depressive disorder associated with subcortical white matter brain changes due to diabetes, cardio-, or cerebrovascular disease	Alexopoulos et al. (1997); Krishnan et al. (2001)
Schizoaffective disorder	Symptoms of schizophrenia (hallucinations, delusions, incoherence, avolition) exist concurrently with major depression or bipolar disorder; symptoms of schizophrenia are present for at least 2 weeks in the absence of a mood disorder	DSM-5
Treatment-resistant depression	Various definitions but generally means at least one, more often two trials of antidepressant therapy at adequate dose and duration have failed to bring about remission	Carney & Freedland (2009)
Positive affect domain (lack thereof, including anhedonia)	Core feature of depressive and obsessive disorders suggested by the Research Domain Criteria initiative, and distinguished from "negative affect" domain, which includes fear, distress, and aggression	Stanislaw et al. (2010)

CHAPTER 2

What Causes Depression in Late Life and What Makes It Difficult to Treat?

Present understanding of the determinants of onset and outcomes of depression remains imperfect. Nonetheless, recommendations for clinical populations and symptomatic individuals are possible and important for practitioners, patients, and their family members. This chapter reviews hypotheses about the cause of depression and obstacles to recovery that have bearing on treatment selection and outcome.

ETIOLOGY

It is popular to ascribe depression to an imbalance in neurochemistry, or a response to overwhelming stress, or an intolerable loss. Each explanation is preferable to the prejudice that someone with a depressive disorder is constitutionally weak. But none approaches the complexity of present etiological hypotheses, whether biomedical or psychosocial or developmental. All the hypotheses are consistent with the stress–vulnerability theory, in which certain individuals are predisposed to the development of depression when stressed (Kendler et al., 2002).These hypotheses related to late-onset depression are discussed in greater detail in what follows.

The Vascular Hypothesis and the Neural Circuitry of Depression

As briefly described in Chapter 1, Krishnan et al. (1993) and Alexopoulos et al. (1997) described major depressive disorders with an onset at age 55 or older that were often associated with changes in the subcortical white matter of the brain previously observed among patients with cardiovascular disease. White matter serves important communication functions. It connects the gray matter processing areas of the brain as well as connecting the lower parts of the brain and body to the cerebral cortex. In approximately one-third of the depressed patients in the above studies, damage to the brain's white matter (appearing as bright periventricular hyperintensities on imaging) and microvascular infarctions (also shown on brain imaging) were found with a frequency not expected for age or severity of cardiovascular disease. Whether the white matter changes played any causative role could not be inferred, but with follow-up it was clear that the benefits of antidepressant medication were lessened when these imaging hyperintensities were present.

Subsequent work examining the functional integrity of neural circuitry reinforced and refined the hypothesis that late-life depression is related to short-circuiting of critical neural pathways. In similar studies of younger patients with treatment-resistant depression, Tao et al. (2013) found an uncoupling of the putative hate circuitry in the brain comprised of the superior frontal gyrus, putamen, and insula. The circuit was originally identified with functional imaging of persons shown pictures of people they hated. In individuals with treatment-resistant depression, this hate circuit showed diminished connectivity without loss of anatomic volume. This suggests a neuroanatomical model for Freud's 1917 observation in *Mourning and Melancholia* that self-loathing distinguishes the sadness of depressive disorders from that of bereavement. What emerges is a functional neuroanatomical model of depression in which frontal–subcortical affect-regulating circuits are disrupted. Dorsal–cognitive and ventral–affective regions mediate the effect.

For example, when shown emotionally charged facial expressions, depressed persons, compared to those without depression, exhibit less activation in regions involved with cognition (dorsal anterior cingulate and dorsolateral prefrontal cortex) and greater activation in regions involved with emotion (the rostral and ventral brain regions, which include the limbic regions: the amygdala, rostral cingulate, and medial prefrontal cortex). Greater white matter damage (indicated by imaging hyperintensities) disrupts brain neural circuits leading to limbic overactivation in which prefrontal cortical structures have diminished capacity to modulate limbic hyperactivity. Whether the effect is due to the global burden of white matter damage or more narrowly defined circuit-specific disruption is unclear. Both discrete and more widespread lesions could have the same effect, provided the critical tracts are impacted. In any event, white matter changes represent a biomarker for depressive illness in which top-down, intellectual management of limbic activity is impaired (Aizenstein et al., 2011).

Because depression contributes to vascular risk factors, including diabetes, hypertension, and smoking, the relationship may be one of both cause and effect. Early-age vascular risk factors lead to structural brain changes, which then predispose the older person to onset of depression in later life. Depression in early life exacerbates vascular risk, leading to white matter changes in late life as well. In summary, the vascular hypothesis of late-onset depression has matured from static observation of associations to a functional neuroanatomical model that approaches causality.

The Inflammation Hypothesis

In the inflammation hypothesis, metabolic rather than vascular processes lead to changes in the function of cognitive and emotion control systems and the hippocampus. These changes are mediated by cytokines, which are polypeptides central to the function of both the peripheral nervous system and the brain's immune system. In the brain, they are produced mainly by astroglia and microglia, although all central nervous system (CNS) cells are capable of cytokine production. Cytokines include interferons (INF), interleukins (IL), colony-stimulating factor (CSF), tumor necrosis factor (TNF), and transforming growth factor (TGF). As the name implies, cytokines transmit information, instructions from one set of cells to another, with consequences potentially protective or pathological. Endothelial cells secrete brain-derived neurotrophic factor (BDNF), which promotes neuronal survival and synaptic plasticity and is reduced in depression. And in animal models advancing age is associated with an increase in the peripheral immune response degraded communication between the peripheral and CNS immune systems, which results in a shift of the CNS into a more pro-inflammatory state. Pro-inflammatory cytokines emanate from adipose tissues, elevate glucocorticoids, and depress the production of neurotrophins and neurogenesis. Interleukins

1 and 6 are associated with obesity and the metabolic syndrome (Song & Wang, 2010).

The dysregulation of the neurotrophic system is posited to underlie the pathogenesis of depression. Exaggerated, prolonged immune reactions may alter neural networks, subtending emotional and cognitive responses similar to behavioral and intellectual changes observed in late-life depression. However, the data suggesting that anti-inflammatory medications have antidepressant effects are scant (Alexopoulos & Morimoto, 2011).

Neurogenesis

The phenomenon of adult neurogenesis, or the ability of the mature brain to generate new neurons, was originally described by Altman and Das (1965) but remained highly controversial for decades. Currently the process whereby neural stem cells migrate into the hippocampus and become fully functioning neurons is seen as critical to our understanding of the major mental illnesses. Inflammatory responses exhibit a close relation to the regulation of neurogenesis (Whitney et al., 2009), for example, stress that induces spikes or prolonged release of corticosterone detrimentally affects adult neurogenesis (Cameron & Gould, 1994). Adult neurogenesis and hippocampal function have major roles in the pathophysiology of anxiety (Revest et al., 2009) and depression (Santarelli et al., 2003). Antidepressant drugs stimulate adult hippocampal neurogenesis (Malberg et al., 2000), and neurogenesis seems to be required for the behavioral effects of antidepressants (Santarelli et al., 2003; for review see Sahay & Hen, 2007). Thus, although neurogenesis may be necessary for recovery, it as yet does not have a recognized role in the etiology of depression (Samuels & Hen, 2011). Neurogenesis is promoted by physical exercise and suppressed by long-term alcohol exposure (Davis, 2008).

Bereavement

Bereavement is a major, predictable life event among older adults. Spousal bereavement is more prevalent among older women, whose survival advantage over their husbands is countered by a greater likelihood of disability, living alone, and nursing home admission. With increased lifespans, older adults more frequently live through the loss of an adult child, even a grandchild. Older persons do not perceive bereavement to be a problem in need of professional attention. Considerable controversy has arisen over DSM-5's dropping of bereavement as an automatic excep-tion to the diagnosis of major depressive disorder (Frances, 2012). How-ever, bereaved older adults are more likely to develop a major depres-sive episode within the year of their loss than younger persons (Zisook, Shuchter, & Sledge, 1994). When crying, sleep disturbance, weight loss, and helplessness are severe, persistent, or disabling, an intervention is warranted. When psychosis or suicidality is present, that intervention may require medication as well.

Two additional conditions related to depression—complicated grief and caregiver burden—are discussed more fully in Chapters 4 and 5, on psychotherapy and psychosocial interventions. Some bereaved persons experience unyielding, extreme preoccupation and longing for their lost loved one and avoid satisfying relations with friends or family. They seem unable to stop grieving. In contrast, caregivers of persons with dementia start grieving long before their loved one's death. Empirically validated interventions for complicated grief and caregiver burden are effective but require more than supportive techniques.

The Stress–Diathesis (Vulnerability) Model

Aspects of the built environment and neighborhood, personality traits, retirement, bereavement, caregiving, trauma, and acutely disabling ill-nesses such as stroke, heart attack, or hip fracture are examples of how factors both intrinsic and extrinsic to the person have an impact on the emergence and persistence of depressive symptoms. For example, the lack of commercial destinations, neighborhood "walkability," and the presence of violence and structural decay are significant contributors to the risk of persistent depressive symptom among older persons, even after controlling for the socioeconomic status of the area. Neighbor-hoods that foster physical activity and social integration may protect against symptoms of depression (Beard et al., 2014).

Personality

Measures of personality domains consistently related to depression across the lifespan include higher neuroticism, lower extroversion, and lower conscientiousness (Hayward et al., 2013). Persons scoring higher on measures of neuroticism are comparatively more reactive autonomi-cally and less stable emotionally (Sato, 2005). They tend to be more anxious, self-conscious, depressive, and vulnerable. Persons scoring lower on the domain of extroversion are characteristically introverted, preferring a quiet, less stimulating environment in keeping with their baseline higher level of autonomic arousal. They are less assertive, tend to avoid stimulation. Persons scoring lower on the domain of conscientiousness portray themselves as less competent, orderly, striving, and self-disciplined. Older adults with this profile of traits do not necessarily experience greater severity of symptoms during a major depressive episode but will be more symptomatic at 3 and 12 months following treatment. As a result, they may require greater assistance with behavioral activation, social support, and problem solving during psychotherapy (Hayward et al., 2013), as described in Chapters 4 and 5.

Retirement

Oliffe et al. (2013) examined the relationship between depression and retirement among older men. For some, retirement meant a loss of self-worth through damage to masculine identities of being a worker and breadwinner. However, retirement could also reflect the endpoint of failed aspirations for wealth and achievement. Depression can also precede retirement as a result of unfulfilling work. Retirement, particularly among men, is a major life event that may reflect as well as provoke vulnerability.

Caregiving

Capistrant, Berkman, and Glymour (2013) examined the onset of depressive symptoms from a representative sample of married older caregivers, defined as those who provided 14 or more hours per week of assistance with basic or instrumental activities of life to a spouse. Elevations in depressive symptoms occurred with the start of caregiving but were not worsened by the duration of caregiving. However, caregiving significantly predicted the incidence of cardiovascular disease. Long-term caregiving doubled the risk of cardiovascular disease onset among whites but not others (Capistrant et al., 2012).

Trauma

Although caregiving and retirement may be perceived as stressful life events, they are not traumatic in the sense of being injurious or life threatening. The relationship between early life trauma and later onset of depression or posttraumatic stress disorder (PTSD) is complicated. The most vulnerable individuals may have succumbed early on, leaving the more resilient among the observed survivors. Conversely, the ongoing aftermath of trauma, be it physical, emotional, or social, may be responsible for the profile of symptoms. Here again the stress–vulnerability model is instructive. Stressful events late in life may uncover or exacerbate the early effects of trauma (Yehuda et al., 1995). The short form of the allele for the serotonin transporter promoter (5-HTTLPR) is thought to mediate the interaction of stress and genetic vulnerability to depression, but its role in late life is largely unexplored. Holocaust survivors appear prominently in the literature of early-life trauma and its manifestations in old age. Their numbers are dwindling, but survivors of armed conflict, domestic abuse, accidental injury, and violence ensure the need for health care providers to be aware of trauma's contribution to depressive disorders.

Advanced Age

In contrast to personality domains and social and environmental stressors, advancing age does not in and of itself confer psychological risk. Indeed, older adults are more resilient (Windle, Markland, & Woods, 2008; Bonanno et al., 2006), less prone to avoid, and less preoccupied with negative, threatening imagery than younger persons with less life experience (Charles, Mather, & Carstensen, 2003; De Raedt, Koster, & Ryckewaert, 2013). As a result, life satisfaction and affective well-being appear to stabilize or even increase during old age, likely due to increased emotional stability and resilience. Older adults tend to recognize their limitations and become more selective in their pursuits, compensating for weaknesses and optimizing strengths, and moderating the stresses of everyday life (Baltes & Baltes, 1990).

WHAT MAKES DEPRESSION DIFFICULT TO TREAT?

Among older adults who develop depression, 23% experience a spontaneous remission (Beekman et al., 2002; Schoevers et al., 2003). For the remainder several characteristics predict difficulty achieving remission with antidepressant therapy. These include greater number of concurrent physical conditions (Dew et al., 2007), depressive symptom severity (Gildengers et al., 2005), higher anxiety (Andreescu et al., 2007), inadequate prior response to antidepressant treatment (Tew et al., 2006), dissatisfaction with social support (Dew et al., 1997), suicidal ideation (Szanto et al., 2001, 2007), a history of recurrent episodes (Driscoll et al., 2005), and the use of concomitant psychotropics such as sleep aids or antianxiety agents (Shelton et al., 2009). Perceived stigma is related to premature discontinuation of treatment among older adults as well (Sirey et al., 2001; see also Table 2.1).

In addition, failure to achieve noticeable reduction in symptom severity within the first 2 weeks of treatment at indicated dosage is a reliable predictor of drug failure weeks later (Mulsant et al., 2006; Dew et al., 2007). Partial response at 6 weeks (with less than 45% reduction in baseline Hamilton depression ratings) is not a favorable prognosis for eventual symptom remission (Andreescu et al., 2008; Mulsant et al., 2006). Although Reynolds et al. (2010) found the addition of interpersonal psychotherapy to bring to remission older adults whose response to escitalopram was less than a 50% reduction in symptom severity, the comparison group in the study received elaborate depression care management that exceeded the vast majority or routine depression care. Nonetheless, slightly fewer than 50% in both groups experienced remission of the depressive episode, confirming the unfavorable prognosis associated with less than full response. Age of onset for the first episode is not a consistent predictor of poor response (Dew et al., 1997; Andreescu et al., 2008; Alexopoulos et al., 1997).

In a longitudinal study of clinically depressed older patients, Bosworth et al. (2002) found that baseline perceived social support was as important as clinical and diagnostic variables in predicting the remission

---

TABLE 2.1. Predictors of Poor Response to Interventions for Depression

- Excess cortical white matter hyperintensities
- Elevated anxiety
- Neuroticism
- Suicidality and psychosis as indicators of both severity and risk of recurrence
- Undisclosed substance abuse
- Intractable social stressors, mistreatment or abuse
- Dementia, executive dysfunction, physical illnesses
- Undetected mania or psychosis
- Inadequate physical activity, suboptimal nutrition (vitamin D_3)
- Overly cautious prescribing
- Inadequate response to prior treatment or history of recurrence
- Ageism (nihilism) among patients and practitioners alike
- Systematic, structural misalignment of resources

of depressive symptoms. Begle et al. (2011) found that emotional, but not physical, abuse was significantly correlated with higher levels of anxiety and depression. Moreover, the correlation remained after controlling for established demographic and social/dependency characteristics. Smits et al. (2008) found that high levels of persistent depressive symptoms were associated with higher levels of anxiety, two or more physical illnesses, functional impairment, lower perception of mastery, lower level of education, and living without a partner.

Among community-residing older adults, declining health and increasing disability are the major predictors of both the emergence and persistence of clinically significant depressive symptoms (Kennedy et al., 1990, 1991). Nearly a quarter (24%) of all noninstitutionalized people ages 65 and older reported their health to be poor. But fully a third of the non-Hispanic black and Hispanic or Latino elders reported poor health. In 2010 only 11% of older adults participated in leisure-time aerobic and muscle-strengthening activities consistent with the federal physical activity guidelines of 2008 (Federal Interagency Forum on Aging-Related Statistics, 2012). Given the relationship between neurogenesis and exercise, lack of physical activity may also contribute to the persistence of depression.

Although white matter changes related to vascular diseases are implicated in the etiology of late-onset depression, gray matter alterations are associated with less favorable outcomes despite adequate dose and duration of antidepressant medication. In the Treatment Outcome in Vascular Depression study (Sheline et al., 2012), in which adults 60 years of age and older were treated with sertraline up to 200 mg daily, smaller hippocampal volumes were associated with slower response to treatment. When extent of white matter hyperintensities and neuropsychological measures were included, cognitive processing speeds in addition to hippocampal volume were the best predictors of slowed response rates over time. Lesser hippocampal volume and frontal pole thickness were associated with failure to achieve remission. Executive function, language, and episodic memory were also significant predictors of rate of response in combination with hippocampal volume, but only processing speed improved the predictive model. This study is all the more noteworthy because persons with cognitive decline were excluded, and the contributions of vascular risk factors were included in the model. In addition, reduction in cognitive processing speed is a well-recognized aspect of healthy aging, but age as well as age of depression onset were controlled in the analyses.

Depression complicated by psychosis is associated with poorer initial response, prolonged time to recovery, and greater residual disability, as well as greater mortality (Meyers et al., 2009). Although alcohol misuse is not always associated with difficult-to-treat depression (Oslin, 2005), unhealthy levels of drinking are not uncommon among older adults. In a national survey Blazer and Wu (2009) found among respondents 65 and older that 13% of men and 8% of women reported at-risk alcohol use, and more than 14% of men and 3% of women reported binge drinking. Among older men dependent upon alcohol but abstinent when initiating sertraline for major depression, as little as 2 days of alcohol intake of any amount during antidepressant treatment significantly reduced the response rate. Among those who relapsed to heavy drinking, the remission rate was cut in half compared to those who remained abstinent (Oslin, 2005). Finally older primary care patients with high levels of depressive symptoms that persisted for a year suffered significantly increased mortality rates over the subsequent 5 years compared to those whose high symptom levels declined more quickly (Bogner et al., 2012).

Executive Dysfunction

Executive function, also called executive cognitive control, is an ensemble of mental processes involved in problem solving, and in planning, sequencing, initiating, and terminating thought and behavior. Executive function includes cognitive flexibility, concept formation, and self-monitoring. Information storage and recall are required for learning and memory. Executive function is required for implementation and task completion. With impaired executive function, instrumental activities of daily living (driving, shopping, accounting, medication management) may exceed the individual's capacity even though memory is relatively normal. One's capacity to exercise self-control and to direct others to meet one's needs becomes diminished. Executive dysfunction was one element in the DSM-IV criteria for the diagnosis of dementia and is a primary criterion even in the absence of memory impairment in DSM-5. Both selective and sustained attention are impaired among depressed adults of any age. However in late-life depression, inhibitory control and sustained effort are preferentially impaired (Alexopoulos et al., 2002). Executive processes are located in prefrontal cortical areas that are separate from those involved in memory and value-based decision making (Gläschera et al., 2012). By clinical implication, a person may value the promise of recovery associated with an intervention but not be able to effect the necessary changes to do so despite being free of memory impairment.

More so than sadness, the more common features of depression associated with executive dysfunction are apathy, cognitive retardation, lack of guilt, poor insight, and excess disability. Inadequate response to antidepressant therapy is often considered an associated feature. Those that do respond are less likely to achieve remission and are more likely to experience relapse as well as to develop dementia (Morimoto et al., 2011). The extent to which executive dysfunction reduces responsiveness to treatment remains to be fully explained, yet most investigators find its contribution significant. A meta-analysis of antidepressant trials conducted in 2009 (McLennan & Mathias, 2010) found that only data from the group led by Alexopoulos (Alexopoulos et al., 2004, 2005a, 2005b; Morimoto et al., 2011) supported the depression–executive dysfunction hypothesis of poor response to antidepressants.

Among executive measures only the Mattis Dementia Rating Scale Initiation/Perseveration subtest and the Stroop color/word interference test predicted poor response. However, subsequent work by Sneed et al. (2010) found poor outcome with citalopram associated with executive dysfunction as evidenced by deficient response inhibition on Stroop's test as well. Citalopram, escitalopram, and nortriptyline are the antidepressants to date that are associated with poor response in depression with executive dysfunction. Royall et al. (2009) argue that sertraline, because of greater dopaminergic activity, reduces executive dysfunction in the context of depression and heart disease. Bupropion has hypothetical appeal for the same reason. However, Weintraub and associates (2010) found sertraline no better than (but as good as) placebo to treat either minor or major depression in patients with Alzheimer's disease in a large randomized controlled trial. Because memory and learning may be preserved despite executive dysfunction, problem-solving therapy may add benefits beyond supportive therapy (Areán et al., 2010). Although impaired cognition is a core feature of major depression, combining donepezil with an antidepressant to prevent recurrence or reduce the risk of dementia may be counterproductive (Reynolds et al., 2011).

Assessing Executive Dysfunction

There are a variety of executive dysfunction measures (see Gläschera et al., 2012), of which the Stroop test is the most highly regarded but also cumbersome to use clinically. The best predictor of remission and poor response to medication was performance on the complex verbal component of the Initiation/Perseveration subscale of the Mattis Dementia Rating scale (Morimoto et al., 2011). It simply asks the patient to describe a 20-item grocery list within 60 seconds. Persons free of executive dysfunction will produce 14 nonduplicate items in 60 seconds. Those using categories to direct their choices (e.g., three dairy items, three vegetables, and so forth) achieve remission from depression earlier. Persons with lower scores were much less likely to experience remission. This, along with other brief assessments of executive dysfunction that are verbally administered and do not require written responses, appear in Table 2.2.

TABLE 2.2. Brief Assessments of Executive Dysfunction

Complex verbal component of the Initiation/Perseveration subscale of the Mattis Dementia Rating Scale (Morimoto et al., 2011)

Ask the subject to generate a 20-item grocery list. Persons free of executive dysfunction will produce 14 nonduplicate items in 60 seconds. Those using categories to direct their choices—for example, three dairy items, three vegetables, and so forth—achieve remission from depression earlier.

Oral Trails Part B (Ricker & Axelrod, 1994)

Ask the subject to count from 1 to 25 and then recite the 26 letters of the alphabet. Persons requiring more than 60 seconds or committing one or more errors on either task do not have sufficient concentration to reliably complete the next step, which is as follows. The subject is asked to pair numbers with letters in sequence (e.g., "1–A, 2–B, 3–C") until "13–M" is reached. More than 2 errors in 13 pairings indicates impairment.

Controlled Oral Word Association Test (Benton, Hamsher, & Sivan, 1994)

With categories beginning with the letter "F," then "A," then "S," ask respondents to fill the category by providing words of three or more letters. For example, correct responses to the category cue "F" would include "fish, foul, fact." This test reflects abstract mental operations related to problem solving, sequencing, and resisting distractions, intrusions, and perseverations. It is considered a "frontal" task, as the organization of words by first letter is unfamiliar, and requires conscious, effortful, systematic organization and the filtering of irrelevant information such as natural taxonomic categories. Persons free of executive dysfunction will produce 10 words in each category within 1 minute. Characteristically, impaired persons experience working memory fatigue, progressively producing fewer words with each category or errors of intrusion from one category to the next.

An online video demonstration of screening older adults for executive dysfunction can be found on the *American Journal of Nursing* website (*http://links.lww.com/A326*).

CONCLUSION

The unifying theme across all the studies reviewed in this chapter is the complex interaction of brain and behavior. The complexity is associated with multiple obstacles to recovery but also multiple avenues of intervention. Specifically, psychotherapies systematically alter the activation of neural circuits in the dorsolateral prefrontal cortex through learning processes that regulate emotional arousal in a top-down fashion. Antidepressants alter activity in regions of the anterior cingulate that are more closely connected to the limbic system. Psychotherapeutic approaches alone, or standard medications alone, may be insufficient to fully remedy the depressive pathology experienced by individuals in whom both systems are dysfunctional (Ressler & Mayberg, 2007). However, we can identify those individuals for whom treatment should be more aggressive, more systematic, and more individualized. The next five chapters present the current range of therapeutic options. Where research support exists, they offer guidelines for which interventions are best suited for which patients.

CHAPTER 3

Pharmacotherapy

L arge-scale studies now offer substantial guidance for the pharma-cotherapy of late-life depression, including which medication to choose when the first choice fails, how to transform partial remission into genuine recovery, and the timing of dose escalation and the final target dose. In addition, the choice of medications for the depression of bipolar disorder as well as depression complicated by psychosis can be based on studies that included significant numbers of older patients. Selecting the best sequence of medications for patients who have not fully responded remains a challenge. There are now research-based algorithms, described in this chapter, to guide the prescribing clinician.

Paradoxically, progress in the science of treatment has highlighted inadequacies and misperceptions in prescriber practice and public expectations. Depression is indeed treatable but requires a more aggressive approach to be treated well. Such an approach includes not just aggressive pharmacotherapy but also active care management, support for both patients and their families, and access to empirically based psychotherapy. The evidence supporting aggressive treatment is described in this chapter. Subsequent chapters cover psychotherapies, other interventions, and the care management platform necessary to realize the full benefits of antidepressant therapy.

GENERAL PRINCIPLES OF PRESCRIBING
FOR OLDER ADULTS

Table 3.1 offers detailed dose recommendations, advantages, and adverse effect profiles for select antidepressants when prescribed for older adults. Several recommendations apply no matter which medication is chosen. First, safety and comorbidity, rather than differences in effectiveness, dictate the choice of antidepressants at any age. Regardless of class, the medication should be started at the lowest dose, then titrated to the recommended level gradually to minimize adverse effects. Patients should be educated about which adverse effects are transient but tolerable (dry mouth, gastrointestinal upset) and which are dangerous (orthostatic hypotension, cardiac arrhythmias). They should also be relieved of the misapprehension that "antidepressants take a month to work." Response trajectory data, discussed later in this chapter, clearly indicate that if the recommended dose is tolerated and if the first choice happens to the right choice, improvement should be seen within days rather than weeks. If the patient is not in some way better early in treatment, a second choice should be offered. It is helpful to tell patient and family at the outset that if the first choice fails or is only partially effective, there are a number of safe and effective alternatives. In practice this means calling the patient 72 hours after the first dose to check on safety and tolerability and, if there are no adverse effects, advising an increase. This safety check will also give patients who were too anxious to initiate treatment an opportunity to voice concerns and avoid further delay. At the next visit, 10 days to 2 weeks later, the patient should be taken to the recommended dose, then seen 10 days to 2 weeks after that. If no benefit is apparent, the medication should be switched. Later in this chapter, I discuss what the research tells us about the selection of agents. First, however, it's helpful to review the limitations of medications used for mood disorders.

Metabolic Limitations (Adverse Reactions)

Adverse effects of antidepressants among older adults may be divided into those that are annoying and those that are dangerous. Most threatening are the dose-related arrhythmia and hypotensive effects of the tricyclic antidepressants and trazodone. Cognitive impairment, dry mouth, and constipation due to the anticholinergic effects of the tricyclics (and to a lesser degree paroxetine) are troublesome but not life threatening.

TABLE 3.1. Select Antidepressants for Older Adults

Generic name	Trade name	Initial dose	Final dose	Amnesia, arrhythmia potential	Hypotensive potential	Sedative potential	Precautions	Advantages
Tricyclics (TCAs)								
nortriptyline	*Pamelor Aventyl*	10–25 mg	25–100 mg	Moderate	Moderate	Moderate	Lower final dose; may be fatal in overdose, glaucoma, prostatic disease, diabetes	Therapeutic window: 50–150 ng/ml
Selective serotonin reuptake inhibitors (SSRIs)								
fluoxetine	*Prozac Prozac Weekly*	10 mg qam 90 mg qwk	20–40 mg	Low	Low	Low	Prolonged T½, nausea, tremor, insomnia, drug interactions	Side effects not life threatening; liquid preparation available; approved for OCD, PD
sertraline	*Zoloft*	25 mg qam	100–200 mg	Low	Low	Low	Nausea, tremor, insomnia	Few drug interactions, liquid concentrate available; FDA approved for OCD, PTSD, social anxiety disorder
paroxetine	*Paxil*	10 mg hs	20–40 mg	Low	Low	Low	Nausea, tremor, drug interactions; reduce dose for renal insufficiency	Mild sedative effect, approved for PTSD, OCD, PD, GAD, social anxiety disorder
citalopram	*Celexa*	10 mg qam	20 mg	Moderate	Low	Low	Nausea, tremor; reduce dose for renal insufficiency; significant arrhythmia risk above 20 mg	Few drug interactions; oral solution available

escitalopram	*Lexapro*	10 mg qam	20 mg	Low	Low	Low	Nausea, tremor; reduce dose for renal insufficiency	Single enantiomer; FDA approved for GAD
vortioxetine	*Brintellix*	5 mg qam	20 mg	Low	Low	Low	Nausea; reduce dose when combined with bupropion, increase dose with carbamazepine	SSRI with 5-HT receptor agonist properties
Selective serotonergic–noradrenergic reuptake inhibitors (SSRIs/SNRIs)								
venlafaxine	*Effexor XR*	37.5 mg qd	225 mg	Low	Low	Low	Mild hypertensive, headache, nausea, vomiting; do not stop abruptly; reduce dose for renal insufficiency	SSRI and SNRI; fewer drug interactions
desvenlafaxine	*Pristiq*	50 mg qam	50–100 mg	Low	Low	Low	Headache, nausea, hypertension, dizziness; reduce dosage in renal insufficiency; few data from older adults	Active metabolite of venlafaxine; narrow dose range
duloxetine	*Cymbalta*	20 mg	40–60 mg	Low	Low	Low	Drug interactions (CYP1A2, CYP2D6 substrate); chronic liver disease, alcoholism, serum transaminase elevation; reduce dose for renal insufficiency or choose other agent	Equally SSRI and SNRI, narrow dose range; FDA approved for neuropathic pain, fibromyalgia, GAD

(continued)

TABLE 3.1. (*continued*)

Generic name	Trade name	Initial dose	Final dose	Amnesia, arrhythmia potential	Hypotensive potential	Sedative potential	Precautions	Advantages
				Monoamine oxidase inhibitors (MAOIs)				
tranylcypromine	*Parnate*	10–20 mg	30–60 mg	Low	Moderate	Low	Life-threatening diet and drug interactions	When depression resists, TCA/SSRI; stimulant; short T½
selegiline	*Emsam patch*	6 mg qd	12 mg qd	Low	Moderate	Low	MAOI type B with life-threatening diet and drug interactions unlikely at prescribed dose	Transdermal patch with less risk of adverse reactions or suicide
				Other antidepressants				
bupropion	*Wellbutrin*	100 mg	100 mg tid	Low	Low	Low	Dopaminergic, noradrenergic, agitation, insomnia, seizures	Anxiolytic; for apathetic depression, when SSRI fails or for combination
	SR	100 mg	150 mg bid					
	XL	150 mg qd	300 mg qd					
trazodone	*Desyrel*	25–50 mg	100–400 mg	Low	High	High	Very sedative, no partial response	For sleep disturbance
vilazodone	*Viibryd*	10 mg hs	40 mg	Low	Low	Low	Nausea, diarrhea; no studies devoted to older adults	Metabolized by CYP3A4; FDA approved for major depressive disorder

mirtazapine	*Remeron Sol-tabs*	7.5 mg	15–45 mg	Low	Moderate	Prolonged T½, dry mouth, weight gain; reduce dose for renal insufficiency	When depression resists, SSRI; sedative, orexigenic
buspirone	*Buspar*	5 mg bid	30 mg	Low	Low	Only for augmentation, not a benzodiazepine substitute	Antianxiety agent with no dependence
L-triiodothyronine	Various T3	25 µg	50 µg	Moderate	Low	Anorexia, arrhythmia, hypertension, only for augmentation	Rapid onset of action
lamotrigine	*Lamictal XR*	25 mg hs	200 mg qd	Moderate	Low	Prolonged T½; appearance of rash calls for immediate cessation; little used in the elderly	Drug interactions unlikely; FDA approved for bipolar depression; chewable and dissolvable dose format available
				Stimulants			
methylphenidate	*Ritalin*	5 mg qam	20 mg bid	Low	Low	Anorexia, insomnia, daytime use only	Quick results; for the frail and apathetic
modafinil	*Provigil*	200 mg qam	400 mg qam	Low	Low	Little used in the elderly; drug interactions	Once daily dosing

Note. T½, half-life; bid, twice daily; tid, three times a day; OTC, over the counter; FDA, U.S. Food and Drug Administration; hs, at bedtime; qam, every morning; qwk, every week; qd, every day; CYP, cytochrome P450; 5-HT, 5-hydroxytryptamine (serotonin); GAD, generalized anxiety disorder; OCD, obsessive–compulsive disorder; PD, panic disorder; PTSD, posttraumatic stress disorder. From Kennedy (2013). Reprinted with permission from the American Geriatrics Society.

The SSRIs are the most frequently prescribed antidepressants. They are safe but hardly a panacea and are associated with weight loss, nausea, diarrhea, agitation, and sexual dysfunction. All the SSRIs may directly induce bradycardia, easy bruising, and hyponatremia due to the syndrome of inappropriate antidiuretic hormone (SIADH), particularly in patients taking diuretics. Hyponatremia is dangerous in part because its onset is unpredictable and insidious. Hyponatremia also occurs with the combined selective serotonergic–noradrenergic reuptake inhibitor (SSRI/SNRI) agents venlafaxine and duloxetine. With increasing doses, some SSRIs also affect dopamine reuptake, which may lead to movement disorders more often encountered with neuroleptics such as haloperidol. These extrapyramidal symptoms include Parkinsonism, akathisia, dystonia, and acute and tardive dyskinesia (Blazer, 2003). To date, citalopram is the only SSRI associated increased risk of arrhythmia due to prolongation of the QT interval (Porsteinsson et al., 2014). Doses above 20 mg should be used with caution.

Also, SSRIs promote osteoporosis at twice the rate of tricyclic antidepressants, and the effect is not explained by the lessened physical activity that so often accompanies depression (Rosen, 2009). Falls may be no less frequent with SSRIs than with tricyclics (Thapa et al., 1998). However, antidepressants as a class are associated prospectively with an increased risk of falls among older community residents, as are opioid receptor agonist analgesics, antipsychotics, and benzodiazepine receptor agonists. Seniors in the Health, Aging and Body Composition Study who used any of these agents had a 50% increased risk of sustaining two or more falls over 12 months. The risk increased more than twofold if more than one agent was used. The risk of falls was progressively elevated as the summated standard daily dose increased from low to moderate to high compared to those not using any of the agents (Hanlon et al., 2009). The addition of bupropion to paroxetine has been found to increase falls in older adults (Joo et al., 2002).

Symptoms following abrupt withdrawal of tricyclic antidepressants have been attributed to anticholinergic rebound. With the introduction of serotonergic reuptake inhibitors, reports have emerged of a serotonergic withdrawal syndrome lasting 2–3 weeks and characterized by light-headedness, insomnia, agitation, nausea, headache, and sensory disturbances. Mood disturbance may also occur. These symptoms are more often reported for the shorter-acting SSRIs (sertraline, paroxetine), but venlafaxine and other SSRIs have also been implicated. These agents should not be stopped abruptly because of the risk of inducing a hypose-rotonergic state (Zajecka, Tracy, & Mitchell, 1997).

In a large cross-sectional UK study of adverse events associated with antidepressant prescriptions among older adults in general practice, SSRIs were associated with greater hazard of all-cause mortality, attempted suicide/self-harm, myocardial infarction, stroke/transient ischemic attack (TIA), falls, and fractures than tricyclics (Coupland et al., 2011). Similarly, SSRIs were more often associated with epilepsy/seizures, adverse drug reactions, and hyponatremia, but not upper gastrointestinal bleeding than tricyclics. Venlafaxine and mirtazapine, grouped as "other antidepressants" in Table 3.1, exhibited greater hazard ratios than either tricyclics or SSRIs for epilepsy, upper gastrointestinal bleed, stroke/TIA, attempted suicide or self-harm, all-cause mortality, and fractures but not falls. These data are noteworthy because of the size of the sample, the finding that nearly one-third of observed, depressed primary care patients, were prescribed a tricyclic antidepressant, and because the hazard ratios were adjusted for age and comorbid physical illnesses. This was an observational trial, not a randomized controlled trial, with results vulnerable to differences in indications. Nonetheless, in an accompanying editorial Hickie (2011) highlighted the need to be more cautious in monitoring the initial weeks of SSRI therapy, a time when adverse reactions are most frequent. Hickie also notes that the unexpected safety of tricyclics seen in this study may have resulted from the use of relatively lower doses. This study is unlikely to make tricyclics more popular among practitioners, but it reinforces the assertion that treatment of depression is more time consuming than once thought.

Limitations Due to Polypharmacy

Drug interactions are a predictable risk for seniors due to the polypharmacy characteristic of so many older depressed adults, but also because of specific metabolic effects of the antidepressants. A number of antidepressants inhibit cytochrome P450 enzymes, which are responsible for the metabolism of the majority of medications. The enzyme CYP3A4 metabolizes 60% of prescribed medications and is moderately inhibited by fluoxetine. Between 8 and 10% of the population lack the enzyme CYP2D6, which is substantially inhibited by paroxetine. A number of analgesics in common use by older patients are also metabolized by

CYP2D6, and duloxetine also interacts with CYP2D6. Inhibition of the P450 system will elevate the levels of anticoagulants, beta-blockers, type 1C antiarrhythmics, and benzodiazepines (Salzman, 2001). Alterations in the P450 system may also affect estrogens and the anticholinesterases. Nonetheless, Mourilhe and Stokes (1998) found a relatively low incidence of serious drug interactions with these agents. Citalopram, escitalopram, and venlafaxine are the least likely to cause problems with other medications as a result of metabolism through the CYP450 system (Blazer, 2003). Clearly it is not so much the patient's age but rather the medications in addition to the antidepressant that indicate the need for caution.

Limitations Due to Prescriber Misconceptions

Roose and Sackeim (2002) refuted two major misperceptions in the care of late-life depression. The first is that older adults take longer to respond to antidepressants, and the second is that antidepressant therapy fails them more frequently than younger persons. On close examination, total response rates and time-to-response do not differ between younger and older adult participants in randomized controlled trials. More important, persons not exhibiting a 30% reduction in symptoms by the first month of therapy experience only a 20% remission rate by 12 weeks. Even allowing for the "start low, go slow" slogan of geriatric prescribing, patients experiencing little benefit from the first weeks of treatment should be switched to another medication. Gildengers et al.'s (2002) data convincingly suggest the practitioner should assess poor response within days rather than weeks of initiating treatment.

An additional problem is the frequency with which depressive symptoms among physically ill persons do not meet criteria for a major depressive disorder. These patients may be transiently symptomatic but fully recover without intervention. Alternatively they may have a dysthymic disorder (persistent depressive disorder in DSM-5), be in partial remission, or have a prodrome heralding major depression. Minor depression is the term most often used to capture this phenomenon, but it has been supplanted by the new terminology of DSM-5 (see Table 1.4). Unfortunately, efforts to find distinguishing characteristics other than past history of major depression have not led to clear guidelines for the clinician's response to minor depression (Lyness et al., 2002; Lavretsky & Kumar, 2002).

Limits of Effectiveness

There are additional difficulties for the patient. The superiority of anti-depressants to placebo may be statistically significant, but the size of the beneficial effect is often rather modest (Gildengers et al., 2002). Nearly two-thirds of patients in their first episode of depression will either not achieve or not sustain a full remission of symptoms following initiation of single-agent antidepressant therapy (Beekman et al., 2002). The delay between initiation of treatment and the patient's perception of benefit remains a problem not only because of pharmacodynamics but also because of the caution with which the antidepressant dose is increased for the older patient. Not surprisingly, one-third of medicated patients do not refill their antidepressant prescriptions after the first month (Mamdani, Parikh, & Austin, 2000). Although the prescription of "heart-safe" SSRI antidepressants by primary care providers has increased markedly, more treatment has not translated into better treatment (Steffens et al., 2000). Lack of follow-up is part of the problem, but it is compounded by the uncertainty patients and clinicians experience when the antidepressant either fails outright or provides only partial relief. Algorithms from primary care and research centers, described later in this chapter, promise to improve older adult treatment by clarifying the alternatives when the first choice proves inadequate.

SELECT AGENTS FOR THE INITIATION OF TREATMENT

Nortriptyline inhibits the reuptake of norepinephrine and is a serotonergic and GABA agonist. It may be effective in doses as low as 10 mg daily and is mildly sedative with a moderate risk of hypotension, arrhythmia, and amnesia. It has mild anticholinergic properties that can be amplified by anticholinergic prescriptions and over-the-counter medications. It possesses a therapeutic window (50–150 ng/ml). Levels below the lower threshold indicate that lack of response is due to too little drug. Levels near the upper threshold indicate that the dose should not be increased due to the risk of toxicity. Increased fluid intake, exercise, and a soluble fiber laxative should also be prescribed to prevent constipation.

Sertraline may be better for lethargic or cognitively impaired, frail, and hypotensive patients. Variations in bioavailability give it a relatively broad dose range. Like sertraline, citalopram and escitalopram are relatively free of drug interactions but have a longer half-life. Paroxetine has more cytochrome CYP2D6-inhibiting properties and is slightly anticholinergic and not a first choice for the older adult. Similarly with fluoxetine, cardiac medications and anticoagulants need to be monitored more closely until the dose of paroxetine is stabilized. Because paroxetine possesses a calming effect, it may be administered at bedtime. Fluoxetine has the dual advantages of being very long-lived and available as a liquid. For those whose medications can be supervised less than daily, fluoxetine may be a superior choice.

For the depression in patients with Parkinson's disease, and especially for the frail patient who cannot tolerate side effects, bupropion may be preferred. Bupropion, a dual dopamine and norepinephrine reuptake inhibitor (Stahl et al., 2004), is free of cardiovascular and cognitive threats and drug interactions. Sustained- and extended-release forms obviate the need for divided dosing. However, bupropion may overstimulate some patients, leaving them agitated and sleepless. Nortriptyline may be superior for depressed patients with Parkinson's disease whose cognition and cardiovascular status are robust (Andersen et al., 1980). When depression complicates vascular dementia or Parkinson's disease, methylphenidate may be prescribed for frail elders who are apathetic, have lost appetite, and are unable to tolerate the nuisance side effects of nortriptyline and SSRIs. Methylphenidate has the advantage of rapidly elevating mood, initiative, and appetite when it is effective (Salzman, 2001).

Venlafaxine is unique among antidepressants in that it mildly elevates blood pressure, and thus should not be administered to persons with hypertension, but has few drug interactions. Nausea, vomiting, and headache are adverse reactions most often occurring when the dose is started too high or advanced too fast. It should not be stopped abruptly. Duloxetine, like venlafaxine, is a combined serotonergic and noradrenergic reuptake inhibitor. It has a convenient narrow dose range and does not elevate blood pressure but is more likely than venlafaxine to interact with other medications. Duloxetine may also be more effective for pain reduction than other agents and is FDA approved for diabetic neuropathy (Goldstein et al., 2004). Vortioxetine is a recently introduced SSRI with 5-HT agonist properties. Although its track record is limited, the study of Katona, Hansen, and Olsen (2012) found it efficacious and well tolerated among older adults with a recurrent episode of major depression. Of note, it was more easily tolerated than duloxetine and improved measures of cognitive performance during the course of treatment.

Mirtazapine is neither anticholinergic nor hypotensive but has a prolonged half-life and is dependent on renal clearance for elimination, requiring caution in persons of advanced age or with reduced kidney function. Mirtazapine may be a first choice for depressed patients whose complaint of insomnia or anorexia is imperative (Karp & Reynolds, 2004). Trazodone is also sedative, and less often associated with weight gain, but associated hypotension limits its safety, making it a rare selection for the older person.

Lamotrigine is an anticonvulsant approved by the U.S. Food and Drug Administration (FDA) for the treatment of bipolar depression. It does not impair sexuality or provoke mania, rarely interacts with other drugs, and is not associated with weight gain. Headache is the most frequently reported adverse event but is not common. Rash develops in one patient per thousand, and its occurrence is both serious and unpredictable (Bowden et al., 2004). Because of prolonged half-life, dose titration should be done more gradually than with other agents, beginning with 25 mg once daily.

ANTIDEPRESSANT ALGORITHMS

The STAGED, STAR*D, PROSPECT, and IMPACT algorithms share nearly identical strategies of treatment initiation and duration, identification of remission and partial response, and exceptional efforts to retain patients in treatment. Each begins with an SSRI possessing a short half-life and little potential for drug interactions or withdrawal syndrome. Fluoxetine, despite being available generically, is absent because its prolonged half-life might interfere with expeditious switching (Fava et al., 2003).

STAGED

The Duke Somatic Treatment Algorithm for Geriatric Depression (STAGED) describes five levels of treatment (Steffens, McQuiod, & Krishnan, 2002). For persons experiencing partial response or no response the choices include either switching to another antidepressant or augmentation with an added agent. By stage four the newer antidepressants have been exhausted, and nortriptyline combined with lithium or with an SSRI is prescribed. STAGED was developed in a university-based psychiatric research setting with ready access to diagnostic procedures and an elite inpatient psychiatric unit not available to the average patient. Indeed, many of the patients suffered recurrent, severe depression. As a result nearly one-quarter of patients studied received electroconvulsive therapy (ECT). But with the full array of treatments available, applied by expert practitioners with aggressive follow-through, the STAGED algorithm gets nearly every patient better and almost two-thirds well.

STAR*D

In STAR*D (Sequenced Treatment Alternatives to Relieve Depression), citalopram was the level one initial choice, followed by a switch to either sertraline, bupropion, or venlafaxine at level two. The first choice for augmentation included bupropion, cognitive therapy, or the antianxiety agent buspirone. Switching to the tricyclic antidepressant nortriptyline or to mirtazapine were options in level three, as well as augmentation with one of the newer antidepressants with lithium. Triiodothyronine (T_3), a medication more familiar to primary care practitioners than monoamine oxidase inhibitors and tricyclics, was also available as an augmentation strategy in level three. Level four included a monoamine oxidase inhibitor (Rush, Travedi, & Fava, 2003). Figure 3.1 displays the best switch and augmentation choices. Table 3.2 details rates of response

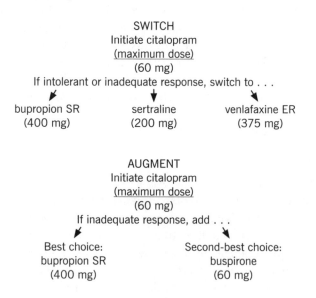

FIGURE 3.1. STAR*D pharmacological "switch" and "augment" algorithms. From Kennedy (2006). Reprinted with permission from *Primary Psychiatry.*

TABLE 3.2. STAR*D Remission, Side Effects, and Intolerance Rates by Medication and Trial Sequence

Trial	Alternative	Medication	Mean dose	Remission	Side Effects	Intolerant
1	None	citalopram	41.8 mg	32.9%	30.2%	8.6%
2	Switch	bupropion SR	282.7 mg	25.5%	31.0%	27.2%
		sertraline	135.5 mg	26.6%	27.1%	21.0%
		venlafaxine XR	193.6 mg	25.0%	35.4%	21.2%
	Augment	citalopram + bupropion	54.8 mg + 267.5 mg	39.0%	23.4%	12.5%
		citalopram + buspirone	55.0 mg + 50.9 mg	32.9%	27.2%	20.6%*
3	Switch	nortriptyline		12.4%	41.1%	NA
		mirtazapine		8.0%	45.3%	NA
	Augment medications from second trial with lithium		859.8 mg	13.2%	34.4%	23.2%
	Augment medications from second trial with T$_3$		45.2 µg	24.7%	29.0%	9.6%***
4	Switch	tranylcypromine	36.9 mg	13.8%	16.7%	41.4%**
	Augment	venlafaxine + mirtazapine	210.3 mg + 35.7 mg	15.7%	24.5%	21.6%

Note. Remission was defined as a score of 5 or less on the QIDS-SR. Side-effects burden was defined as moderate to marked impairment. NA, not available. From Kennedy (2006). Reprinted with permission from *Primary Psychiatry*.

*$p < .05$ compared to citalopram + bupropion; **$p < .05$ compared to venlafaxine + mirtazapine; ***$p < .05$ compared to agents augmented with lithium.

and adverse reactions through level four. I come back to this algorithm, and the research behind it, later in this chapter.

PROSPECT

The algorithm developed by investigators with the Prevention of Suicide in Primary Care Elderly: Collaborative Trial (PROSPECT) incorporated existing treatment guidelines for depression treatment in primary care settings. Citalopram was the first choice, but if the patient was medicated with another antidepressant at substandard dose or duration, that medication was "optimized" to the recommended dose for 12 weeks before considering either switch or augmentation. Of note, the first scheduled dose escalation was 72 hours after the initiation of treatment. Nonresponders could be offered nortriptyline. However, the use of a monoamine oxidase inhibitor or augmentation for nonresponders was considered beyond the scope of primary care providers. Lithium and nortriptyline, as well as the newer antidepressants, could be used to augment treatment for partial responders (Mulsant et al., 2001a).

IMPACT

The antidepressant algorithm from the Improving Mood: Promoting Access to Collaborative Treatment (IMPACT) study in primary care also started with an SSRI, to be followed by a switch to a different class of medication for nonresponders. In the treatment manual Unützer (1999) recommended a rapid switch between SSRIs with minimal time for tapering. However, caution should be exercised when switching between an SSRI and a tricyclic or augmenting the SSRI with a tricyclic because the SSRI may elevate the tricyclic level.

THE PITFALL OF TREATING
THE MOST PROMINENT COMPLAINT

Mulsant et al. (2014) in a painstaking systematic review of randomized controlled trials, observational studies, and the most recent published guidelines on treatment for geriatric depression (Buchanan et al., 2006), categorically reject the notion that the choice of antidepressant be based on the most salient complaint of the depressed older adult. This practice has typically meant that a more sedative agent be offered when the depressed patient complains of insomnia, or a more activating antidepressant when apathy or fatigue are more prominent. The authors acknowledge that this is common clinical practice but contradicted by empirical evidence. They argue for a four step algorithm with each step requiring 6 weeks but with a range from 4 to 8 weeks duration. The first step offers escitalopram with alternatives of sertraline or duloxetine. Step two is taken when there is minimal or no response and switches to duloxetine with venlafaxine or desvenlafaxine as alternatives. Should there be minimal or no response then, in step three nortriptyline is offered with bupropion as the alternative. However if a partial response results from steps two or three, lithium or a second generation atypical antipsychotic (aripiprazole, quetiapine) would be added to augment the response. Alternatives for augmentation include combining an SSRI with an SNRI (e.g., escitalopram or sertraline with duloxetine), or adding mirtazepine or bupropion. The choices of medications and duration of trials are based on simplicity, minimal drug–drug interactions, and less likelihood of adverse reactions. The authors also note that for partial responses augmentation is preferred over switching agents in order not to sacrifice the existing response even if it is partial. They also note that atypical antipsychotics are more easily monitored than lithium but also associated with increased mortality among older adults.

WHEN TWO ANTIDEPRESSANTS ARE BETTER THAN ONE

"Augmentation" is the addition of one antidepressant to ongoing therapy with another. It is more common than "combination" therapy, which is starting treatment with two agents. However, combined therapy with two serotonergic antidepressants (e.g., sertraline in the morning plus trazodone at night), an antidepressant with valproic acid, or an antidepressant combined with thyroid replacement therapy is increasing in frequency.

Prior to the publication of the STAR*D findings, polls of psychopharmacologists showed that the addition of bupropion or methylphenidate was the first choice to augment SSRI treatment. Augmentation with mirtazapine, olanzapine, and buspirone was less preferred (Fava, Mischoulon, & Rosenbaum, 1998). Augmentation strategies are generally employed when the patient has achieved only partial remission after no less than 6 weeks at an adequate dose with a single antidepressant or remained severely symptomatic after trials of single medications from differing classes (Fava et al., 2003; Rush et al., 2003). The use of lithium to augment the response to antidepressants is problematic in the elderly because of reduced renal function and structural brain changes. In addition, lithium may be toxic despite a therapeutic level within the normal range in the older patient. The most cautious approach of once daily dosing is also the most convenient.

Examining the STAR*D Augmentation Guidelines

Reports from STAR*D offer an enormous advance in the effort to empirically direct both switch and augmentation protocols and as such deserve close review (Trivedi et al., 2006a, 2006b; Rush et al., 2006; Fava et al., 2006; McGrath et al., 2006; Nierenberg et al., 2006a; DeGruy, 2006). The results can be applied, with minor reservations, to older adults with depressive disorders (Kennedy, 2006). At the outset the investigators sought a sample of "real world" patients seeking care and making choices at clinical centers rather than those who might be recruited through advertisements or public service announcements. The study occurred in primary care and mental health care sites including both public and private outpatient venues. There were 2,876 persons in the sample; 37.9% were cared for by primary care providers who also treated their depression. Most had comorbid general medical conditions. The most common comorbid psychiatric condition was an anxiety disorder. More than three-quarters met criteria for recurrent depression and nearly one in five reported one or more suicide attempts. One would expect this prevalence of recurrent depression would be associated with reduced remission rates, which was precisely what STAR*D was designed to address. Excluded were persons with depression complicated by psychosis, dementia, or bipolar disorder. Three-quarters of the patients were Caucasians, 17.6% were African Americans, and 13% were Latino. Thus, the racial and ethnic character of the sample resembled that of older Americans. And as with the majority of older adults treated for depression, a substantial number of STAR*D participants received depression care from primary providers. However, persons over the age of 75 were excluded, and most of those included were not experiencing their first episode of depression.

Depression severity measures included the Quick Inventory of Depressive Symptomatology—Self-Report (QIDS-SR) and the Hamilton Depression Rating Scale (HAM-D). The HAM-D is the most widely used measure of depression severity and considered the gold standard for antidepressant trials. The QIDS-SR was developed for ease of patient self-report. Responses are based more on symptom severity than symptom frequency. The QIDS-SR was administered by research technicians every other week with results entered into a web-based treatment monitoring system, which allowed clinical coordinators to guide physicians in antidepressant dosing when symptoms remained elevated and side effects were negligible. The primary outcome of interest was remission based on a HAM-D score representing a virtual absence of depression symptoms and thereby minimal risk of relapse. Both the QIDS-SR to direct therapy and the HAM-D to define outcomes were administered over the telephone.

STAR*D used innovative procedures to allocate patients who did not experience remission with the first antidepressant trial to a series of alternatives. Because each alternative was presumed to be equally effective in the absence of data indicating otherwise, participants were allocated to predetermined alternatives via equipoise-stratified randomization. This meant that all who did not achieve a QIDS-SR-defined remission with citalopram initially were then encouraged to accept any of seven potential alternatives. These included simply switching to another antidepressant, augmentation with an additional agent, and/or cognitive-behavioral psychotherapy. Patients, as in routine clinical practice, could decline one or more alternatives, in which case they were randomized to the remaining "acceptability strata." Table 3.2 displays the various alternatives and levels employed in the trials. All participants were given citalopram initially at 20 mg per day, which was raised to 40 mg per day by week 4, up to a maximum 60 mg per day by week 6. Treatment visits were to occur at 2, 4, 6, 9, and 12 weeks. After the initial trial based on guideline-defined dose and duration of citalopram, all who did not achieve remission were encouraged to enter the equipoise-stratified randomized trial. Patients could discontinue citalopram and move to the next trial before 12 weeks by choice of if they could not achieve or tolerate the optimal dose due to adverse reactions. Persons remaining symptomatic by QIDS score criteria after 9 or 12 weeks despite maximal dose were also offered a subsequent trial.

Table 3.2 also displays the pharmacological profile of the antidepressants used in the trials. Bupropion and buspirone were taken twice daily, all others once daily. Dietary precautions were required for the monoamine oxidase inhibitor tranylcypromine. Single medications chosen for switch monotherapy after citalopram included sertraline, venlafaxine, and bupropion, each designed to answer a different clinical question. Citalopram and sertraline are SSRIs; venlafaxine shows serotonergic and noradrenergic reuptake inhibition (SNRI). Bupropion has both noradrenergic and serotonergic properties but is neither an SSRI or SNRI. As a result the choices for the early monotherapy trials operated by different mechanisms of action with little difference in safety or ease of administration. Medications chosen for later monotherapy trials included nortriptyline, mirtazapine, and tranylcypromine, each with mechanisms of action differing from the prior alternatives but burdened by a more troublesome profile of adverse effects. The monoamine oxidase inhibitor tranylcypromine is associated with life-threatening diet and drug interactions and is unlikely to be prescribed by primary care physicians.

Agents used for augmentation (bupropion, buspirone, mirtazapine) also possessed different mechanisms of action not duplicating SSRIs or SNRIs. Similarly the inclusion of lithium and T_3 for augmentation reflected different theoretical mechanisms not incompatible with any monotherapy or augmentation combinations from the first or second trials. In addition, lithium and T_3 were the most widely studied medications used to augment the effects of antidepressants prior to STAR*D. Dosing and safety monitoring for T_3 was thought to be more familiar to primary care providers, whereas lithium would be more familiar to psychiatrists.

Table 3.2 provides mean dose of medication at the end of each trial along with percentages of marked to moderately burdensome adverse effects. Also included is the percentage of patients who could not tolerate the medication due to adverse effects or discontinued the trial prior to an adequate duration due of lack of improvement. Within the initial citalopram trial, participants with longer index episodes of depression, more concurrent psychiatric disorders, more general medical disorders, and lower baseline function and quality of life experienced lower remission rates. Age was not associated with less likelihood of remission. Of those who achieved remission, 40.3% required 8 weeks of citalopram to do so. Of those who did not experience remission despite being able to tolerate nearly 60 mg of citalopram, an additional third experienced remission when bupropion or buspirone was added. Bupropion was the better of the two choices due to tolerability. Of persons who did not achieve remission with citalopram, one in four remitted simply by switching to sertraline, bupropion SR, or venlafaxine XR. However,

56% of this group could not tolerant citalopram's adverse effects. As a result, the choice of the seemingly more desirable augmentation was not possible.

For patients not well after two antidepressant trials of either mono-therapy or augmentation, switching to nortriptyline, mirtazapine, or tranylcypromine or adding venlafaxine to mirtazapine brought approximately one in eight to remission. Without a placebo control it is possible that one in eight was no better than the spontaneous remission rate of the natural history of recurrent depression. In contrast, of persons who remained symptomatic but tolerated citalopram plus bupropion SR or venlafaxine XR or monotherapy with sertraline, bupropion SR, or venlafaxine XR, nearly one in four reached remission with the addition of T_3. And T_3 was significantly better tolerated than lithium. In summary, STAR*D demonstrates that if the first SSRI cannot be tolerated or proves inadequate, the second can be expected to be reasonably effective. If the first SSRI is tolerated but does not bring about remission, the addition of bupropion will be both safe and effective. Simple protocols of switching or augmentation as shown in Figure 3.1 should achieve remission rates of 60 to better than 70% even when most of the patients have recurrent depressive disorder. And finally, STAR*D suggests that augmentation with T_3 is a safer choice than lithium or switching to the riskier nortriptyline, mirtazapine, or tranylcypromine.

BIPOLAR DEPRESSION

Strakowski (2007) has characterized the lack of data on bipolar depression by noting that nine agents are approved by the FDA for the treatment of mania, but only two (quetiapine and the olanzapine/fluoxetine combination) are approved specifically for bipolar depression. Table 3.3 displays the agents suitable for older adults to stabilize mood in bipolar depression, with doses, precautions, and therapeutic levels. Table 3.4 lists agents to stabilize mood or combat mania in late life. Ziprasidone and chlorpromazine were omitted due to cardiovascular hazards despite FDA approval. As seen in the tables, several medications are approved for episodes of "mixed" mania and depression. Historically, off-label use of antidepressants for bipolar disorder has been common. However, a number of studies suggest that antidepressants may be counterproductive.

TABLE 3.3. Agents Used to Stabilize Mood in Bipolar Depression

Generic name	Trade name	Initial dose	Final dose	Sedative potential	Precautions	Advantages
Lithium compounds						
lithium carbonate controlled release	Eskalith Eskalith CR Lithobid	300 mg qd 450 mg qd 300 mg qd	300 mg tid 450 mg bid 300 mg tid	Low	Renal clearance is sole route of elimination; toxicity may appear below therapeutic range; mild tremor is a benign universal side effect, but not when excessive or combined with ataxia; polyuria, polydipsia may be signs of diabetes insipidus; nausea, vomiting are signs of toxicity; risk of hypothyroidism, renal impairment	FDA approved for acute and maintenance therapy of mania in bipolar disorder; lowers risk of suicide; therapeutic level: 0.6–1.0 mEq/liter
Antipsychotics						
olanzapine	Zyprexa Zydis (oral dissolving)	2.5 mg	15 mg	Moderate	Slightly anticholinergic as dose increases, weight gain, metabolic syndrome, diabetes	FDA approved for acute manic and mixed bipolar I episodes
olanzapine/ fluoxetine	Symbyax	6 mg/ 25 mg	12 mg/25 mg		Few data on use in the elderly	FDA approved for bipolar depression
quetiapine	Seroquel	25 mg	750 mg	Moderate	Sedation, weight gain, metabolic syndrome, diabetes, arrhythmia	FDA approved for acute manic and bipolar I and II depression; sedative; fewer extrapyramidal symptoms, tardive dyskinesia
risperidone	Risperdal	0.25 mg	6 mg	Low	Extrapyramidal symptoms likely at doses above 2 mg, weight gain,	FDA approved for acute manic and mixed bipolar

Generic	Brand	Starting dose	Target dose	Weight gain risk	Side effects/monitoring	Indications
					metabolic syndrome, diabetes, reports of stroke	I episodes
aripiprazole	*Abilify*	2.5 mg	15 mg	Low	Prolonged T½; may produce agitation at high doses due to D2 dopamine receptor agonist activity	FDA approved for acute manic and mixed bipolar I episodes, antidepressant augmentation

Anticonvulsants

Generic	Brand	Starting dose	Target dose	Weight gain risk	Side effects/monitoring	Indications
divalproex sodium extended release delayed release	*Depakote* *Depakote ER* *Depakote DR*	250 mg bid 250 mg hs 125 mg hs	1,000 mg bid 1,000 mg hs 500 mg hs	Moderate	Delayed onset of action, drug interactions, gastrointestinal upset, tremor, weight gain, edema, thrombocytopenia, sedation; complete blood count and chemistries at baseline, then every 6 months; inhibits hepatic enzymes and increases other drug levels; hepatotoxicity, pancreatitis; reduce dose for renal insufficiency	FDA approved for acute manic and mixed bipolar I episodes, better tolerated than carbamazepine; therapeutic level 50–100 µg/ml
carbamazepine	*Tegretol* *Epitol* *Equetro (extended release)*	100 mg bid 100 mg hs	500 mg bid 800 mg hs	Moderate	Delayed onset of action, drug interactions, dizziness, unsteady gait, anemia; complete blood count and chemistries at baseline, then every 6 months; enhances CYP activity and decreases other drug levels	FDA approved for acute manic and mixed bipolar I episodes; therapeutic level 4–12 µg/ml
lamotrigine	*Lamictal*	25 mg hs	100 mg bid	Low	Headaches, prolonged T½, appearance of rash calls for immediate cessation	FDA approved for bipolar I depression to prevent recurrence, does not alter CYP activity

Note. Abbreviations as in Table 3.1.

55

TABLE 3.4. Agents Used to Stabilize Mood or Combat Mania in Late Life

Generic name	Trade name	Initial dose	Final dose	Sedative potential	Precautions	Advantages
Benzodiazepine						
clonazepam	*Klonopin*	0.25 mg bid	2 mg bid	Moderate	Prolonged T½, falls, controlled substance, may exacerbate aggression or confusion in dementia; sedation	Rapid onset, fewer drug interactions, sedation
Lithium compounds						
lithium carbonate	*Eskalith*	300 mg qd	300 mg tid	Low	Renal clearance is sole route of elimination; toxicity may appear below therapeutic range; mild tremor is a benign universal side effect, but not when excessive or combined with ataxia; nausea, vomiting are signs of toxicity; risk of hypothyroidism	FDA approved for bipolar disorder, patient preference, lowers risk of suicide; therapeutic level: 0.6–1.0 mEq/liter
	Eskalith CR	450 mg qd	450 mg bid			
controlled release	*Lithobid*	300 mg qd	300 mg tid			
Antipsychotics						
olanzapine	*Zyprexa* *Zydis* (oral dissolving)	2.5 mg	15 mg	Moderate	Slightly anticholinergic as dose increases, weight gain, IM form available	FDA approved for acute mania, bipolar depression
quetiapine	*Seroquel*	25 mg	750 mg	Moderate	Slit-lamp exam for cataracts	FDA approved for mania, sedative, fewer extrapyramidal symptoms, tardive dyskinesia

risperidone	Risperdal Consta injection	0.25 mg 25 mg q 2 wk	6 mg	Low	Extrapyramidal symptoms likely at doses above 2 mg, high potency, reports of stroke	Available in liquid form; FDA approved for acute mania
aripiprazole	Abilify	5 mg	15 mg	Low	Prolonged T½, may produce agitation at high doses due to D2 dopamine receptor agonist activity	FDA approved for acute mania, antidepressant augmentation

Anticonvulsants

Divalproex sodium extended release delayed release	Depakote Depakote ER Depakote DR	250 mg bid 250 mg hs 125 mg hs	1,000 mg bid 1,000 mg ha 500 mg hs	Moderate	Delayed onset of action, drug interactions, gastrointestinal upset, tremor, weight gain, edema, thrombocytopenia; complete blood count and chemistries at baseline, then every 6 months; inhibits hepatic enzymes and increases other drug levels; hepatotoxicity, pancreatitis; reduce dose for renal insufficiency	FDA approved for acute mania, better tolerated than carbamazepine; therapeutic level: 50–100 µg/ml; putative neuroprotective effect
carbamazepine	Tegretol Epitol Equetro (extended release)	100 mg bid 100 mg hs	500 mg bid 800 hs	Moderate	Delayed onset of action, drug interactions, dizziness, unsteady gait; complete blood count and chemistries at baseline, then every 6 months; enhances CYP activity and decreases other drug levels	FDA approved for bipolar disorder; therapeutic level: 4–12 µg/ml
lamotrigine	Lamictal	25 mg hs	400 mg qd	Moderate	Prolonged T½; appearance of rash calls for immediate cessation	FDA approved for bipolar depression, does not alter CYP activity, drug interactions unlikely

Note. Abbreviations as in Table 3.1.

Sachs et al. (2007) sought to determine whether adding an antidepressant to a mood stabilizer (lithium or an antiepileptic) improved symptoms of bipolar depression without increasing the risk of treatment-emergent mania. They were also interested in the durability of recovery, defined as no less than 8 weeks virtually free of depressive symptoms. Patients received a mood stabilizer plus either an antidepressant or placebo in random fashion. Rates of mania or hypomania were less among the mood-stabilizer-only group. Similarly, somewhat more than a quarter of those in the mood-stabilizer-only group achieved a durable recovery, compared to somewhat less than a quarter of those who received an antidepressant as well. The differences were not statistically significant. Adding an antidepressant conveyed no advantage above that observed for a mood stabilizer alone.

This finding mirrors that of Nemeroff et al. (2001), who found that once the patient's lithium level had reached 0.8 mEq/liter, neither imipramine nor paroxetine conveyed any additional benefits to the treatment of bipolar depression. Nierenberg et al. (2006b) examined 66 bipolar patients experiencing a current major depressive episode who had not responded to adequate doses of mood stabilizers and at least one antidepressant. The patients were randomly assigned to inositol, lamotrigine, or risperidone. The primary outcome was a durable recovery period as defined above. Pairwise comparisons did not reach statistical significance, and the investigators were not blinded to medication choice. The recovery rate, level of depressive symptoms, Clinical Global Impression, and Global Assessment of Functioning all favored lamotrigine. Even so, somewhat less than one-quarter of the lamotrigine group achieved a durable recovery.

Leverich et al. (2006) randomized patients with bipolar depression to receive a mood stabilizer plus either bupropion, sertraline, or venlafaxine. Depending on whether or not there was a past history of mania, from 20 to 35% of patients experienced either treatment-emergent mania or hypomania. In fewer than a quarter of patients was there a sustained response to the antidepressant without the emergence of mania or hypomania. The highest risk was found with venlafaxine, the lowest with bupropion. Goldberg et al. (2007) conducted a similar study among bipolar patients with mixed mania and depression. They found the addition of an antidepressant did not speed recovery. After 3 months of follow-up, significantly higher mania symptom severity was associated with antidepressants compared to mood stabilizers alone.

In summary, the consensus based on expert opinion (Strakowski, 2007; Nierenberg et al., 2006b), guidelines (Hirschfeld, 2005; Hilty et al., 2006), and the Systematic Treatment Enhancement Program for Bipolar Disorder (STEP-BD) reports (Leverich, 2006; Goldberg et al., 2007), is that mood stabilizers are preferable both for acute and maintenance treatment of late-life bipolar depression. Figure 3.2 displays an algorithm based on reports of Calabrese et al. (1999), Hilty et al. (2006), and Dolder, Depp, and Jeste (2007). The prescribing pathway is characterized as much by off-label practice as it is by FDA-approved indications. Beyond the initial prescription of either lithium or lamotrigine, next steps are dictated by the patient's symptom profile. For depressive episodes of both bipolar type I and II with relatively less history of mania, the antidepressant bupropion is a reasonable addition. However, when the presentation is characterized by mixed symptoms or more frequent episodes of mania, an atypical antipsychotic or a second mood stabilizer is preferable (Thase et al., 2006; Perlis et al., 2006b). Simply based on the adverse effects profile and likelihood of drug interactions, lamotrigine is preferable to lithium, divalproex, and carbamazepine for

Primary mood stabilizer:
lamotrigine or lithium
↓
Attain adequate dose or therapeutic level
↓
For inadequate response, add medication depending on the following:

Depressive episode		Mixed episode
Mania rare	Mania frequent	Mixed mania
Not rapid cycling	Rapid cycling	and depression
No history of antidepressant-induced mania	History of antidepressant-induced mania	
↓	↓	↓
bupropion or SSRI, not tricyclic, not SNRI	lamotrigine valproate olanzapine lithium	valproate olanzapine risperidone aripiprazole lithium

FIGURE 3.2. Pharmacotherapy of bipolar depression and mixed depression with mania. From Kennedy (2008). Reprinted with permission from *Primary Psychiatry.*

older adults. Nonetheless, lithium has a longer history of use than any other mood stabilizer for older persons. Shulman (2010) warns against abandoning its proven benefits. He suggests that prescriber practices and lack of guidelines for the use of lithium in late life rather than intrinsic properties may account for its status. For patients so severely disturbed that they refuse life-saving medications (insulin, antiarrhythmics) or cannot control suicidal intent or aggressive outbursts, electroconvulsive therapy is an effective option (Lisanby, 2007; Sackeim & Prudic, 2005). However, there are reports of manic reactions to ECT among older persons (Serby, 2001). Particularly for older patients, practitioners will exhaust alternatives before suggesting this treatment.

Psychotic Depression

The evidence directing choice of pharmacotherapy when psychosis complicates depression in late life is only now emerging. Mulsant et al. (2001b) randomized 52 patients, mean age of 72, with a major depressive episode and psychotic features to nortriptyline plus perphenazine or nortriptyline plus placebo. At the outset all were openly treated with nortriptyline, with the dose titrated to 50–150 ng/ml (target 100 ng/ml). Those not responding within 2 weeks were then administered either placebo ($n = 19$) or perphenazine ($n = 17$) in a randomized double-blind protocol. The placebo or perphenazine doses were titrated to a maximum dose of 24 mg per day until either a therapeutic response or extrapyramidal effects were observed. The final mean dose of perphenazine was 18.9 mg per day. After a mean of 9 weeks of combined therapy, only 50% of those receiving nortriptyline plus perphenazine and 44% receiving nortriptyline plus placebo achieved a categorical response. There were no statistically significant differences between the two groups in terms of depression severity as measured by the HAM-D or the psychoticism subscale of the Brief Psychiatric Inventory. Although the response rate among patients with a Mini-Mental State Examination score of 27 or above was twice that of those with a score below, the difference was not significant. Moreover, of the 36 patients randomized, only 5 reached the target dose of perphenazine and only 30 completed the study.

The authors concluded that the modestly beneficial response rates did not outweigh the potential toxicity of a tricyclic antidepressant combined with a typical antipsychotic. They also speculated that mild cognitive impairment and the short period of treatment might account for the poor results. They concluded that atypical antipsychotics and alternative antidepressants either singly or in combination might achieve better results but that ECT should be offered promptly for patients not responding, rather than attempting prolonged serial medication trials. ECT is effective for depression complicated by psychosis (American Psychiatric Association, 2000; Lisanby, 2007) and is often considered the treatment of choice due to adverse events and poor response rates associated with single-drug or combined antidepressant and antipsychotic therapy (Meyers et al., 2001). Yet few patients and their family members will accept ECT without having exhausted alternatives. As a result the need for better predictors of successful pharmacotherapy is critical.

The Study of Pharmacotherapy of Psychotic Depression (STOP-PD) was designed to have sufficient sites and participants of an extended age range to address limitations of prior studies (Meyers et al., 2006). For diagnostic precision, the investigators excluded persons with schizoaffective disorder, dementia, body dysmorphic disorder, and obsessive–compulsive disorder even if they met criteria for psychotic depression. To examine the effect of age on treatment responsiveness as well as tolerance, participants were stratified by age such that the number of persons ages 18–59 would nearly equal the number ages 60 and older. The investigators also sought to study the relationship between global impairment generally and executive dysfunction specifically as predictors of poor response. Executive cognitive dysfunction was measured with the Stroop Color-Word Test and the Initiation/Perseveration subtest of the Mattis Dementia Rating Scale. For a global measure of cognitive impairment they chose the Mini-Mental State Examination.

To extend the period of treatment beyond the observations of prior studies, a 12-week acute phase of treatment was followed by a 12-week stabilization phase. In the acute phase, participants were randomized to either olanzapine plus placebo or sertraline plus olanzapine initially. Three outcome measures were chosen for the 12-week acute phase. These included (1) partial remission, defined as a 30% reduction in symptoms to a score no higher than 17 from the baseline HAM-D, and (2) full remission, defined as a score of less than 10 on the HAM-D. Participants achieving neither of these outcomes and those who continued to have hallucinations or delusions despite meeting Hamilton criteria for partial or full remission were considered to have reached the third outcome of nonremission. For the following 12-week stabilization phase, those in partial remission who had received sertraline plus olanzapine were randomized to augmentation with either lithium or placebo. Those in partial remission who had initially been given placebo plus olanzapine received augmentation with sertraline plus either placebo or lithium. This allowed a comparison of the benefits of adding lithium when a partial remission occurred for persons previously treated with combined sertraline plus olanzapine, compared to the addition of sertraline for those treated previously with olanzapine only.

The dosing protocol started with olanzapine 5 mg each evening and/or sertraline 50 mg each morning. Doses were increased every 3 to 7 days up to a target of 15 mg olanzapine and/or 150 mg sertraline based on tolerability and response. Patients who remained symptomatic after reaching target doses could receive up to 200 mg of sertraline and 20 mg olanzapine. If the medication dose were reduced as a result of intolerance and the patients remained symptomatic, they were rechallenged with the higher dose at a later date. Overall remission was achieved in 40% of all patients randomized. But of those who completed the study and received the combination of sertraline plus olanzapine, 67% experienced remission. The chances of remission with combination therapy were substantially and significantly better than with sertraline alone. The average end-of-study daily doses were more than 12 mg of olanzapine and nearly 150 mg of sertraline (Meyers et al., 2009). The average age of participants was 72 years. Remission rates were comparable for those above and below 60 years of age. Weight gain was frequent but more prevalent among younger participants. The effects of physical illness, executive dysfunction, global cognitive impairment, and augmentation with lithium have yet to be reported. In addition, the profile of persons least likely to respond or to tolerate sertraline combined with olanzapine and who should be offered ECT early rather than later remains to be determined.

CONCLUSION

Data emerging since 2005 indicate the need for a much more aggressive approach to the pharmacotherapy of late-life depression. Practitioners should first help the patient achieve the right dose more rapidly and, second, switch or augment less than fully effective medications over a matter of weeks, not months. For the depression of bipolar illness, a mood-stabilizing antiepileptic with or without an atypical antipsychotic should be used rather than an antidepressant. To combat depression complicated by psychosis, combining an SSRI with an atypical antipsychotic is superior to an SSRI alone, but the doses may need to be substantial. And to be maximally effective, the array of treatments offered should include ECT when other measures fail or the condition has become life threatening.

A key aspect of the effectiveness of the PROSPECT and IMPACT studies was the use of care management platforms that incorporated mental health specialists into primary care settings and provided access to empirically based psychotherapy and support for both patients and their family members. The care management programs used in these studies are discussed in more detail in Chapters 8 and 9. The type of aggressive care described in this chapter will remain an ideal rather than a reality without such programs. To be broadly effective, antidepressant medication must be enhanced with techniques meant to guide the prescriber, sustain the patient, ensure recovery, and prevent recurrence. If more treatment continues to mean only more prescriptions, the promise of antidepressants will remain unfulfilled. Without including disease management and psychotherapy, we will never be able to ensure that old age and depression are the rarest of companions.

CHAPTER 4

Effective Psychotherapies

Advances in pharmacotherapy have slowed, but evidence supporting the benefits of psychotherapy in primary care, mental health settings, over the Internet, and via telephone continues to expand. Familiarity with psychotherapeutic techniques is crucial to effective, efficient care wherever the provider practices and whatever the age of the patient.

A government-commissioned review of interventions for depression found good evidence that psychotherapeutic approaches are effective among older adults in primary care settings (O'Connor et al., 2009). Yet it remains uncertain which psychotherapy should be directed at which type of depression (Wilson, Mottram, & Vassilas, 2008; Scogin et al., 2005; Gallagher-Thompson & Thompson, 1995; Karasu, 1986) and under what circumstances psychotherapy may be recommended without an antidepressant (Thompson et al., 2001; Areán & Cook, 2002; Pinquart, Duberstein, & Lyness, 2006; Hanson & Scogin, 2008). In Areán's opinion (Agronin, 2009), CBT may be preferred to help older depressed adults regulate emotion. Problem-solving therapy (PST) may be better when executive dysfunction complicates depression and interpersonal psychotherapy (IPT) better for depression wrapped in transitional stresses like grief. When limited to studies of older adults, there are few differences in outcomes when CBT is compared head to head with psychodynamic treatment (Wilson et al., 2008).

In addition, the evidence base supporting empirically validated therapies, though sufficient, is limited compared to that which supports antidepressants, particularly for older adults. Nonetheless, the effect size of 0.78 for psychosocial interventions in geriatric depression compared to placebo or no intervention obtained from meta-analyses contrasts favorably with that for antidepressant medication (Scogin & McElreath, 1994; Pinquart et al., 2006). Even a more conservative estimate of effect size suggests that psychotherapy for depression is significantly beneficial (Cuijpers et al., 2010). Effect sizes for psychotherapies provided to patients with comorbid physical illnesses range from small for PST to large for behavioral activation. Cognitive therapy, CBT, and IPT demonstrated moderate effect sizes (Whooley, 2012). Thus neither age nor physical illness should be seen as obstacles to psychotherapy provided mobility, morbidity, or frailty do not render the prescription impractical. CBT by telephone for depressed primary care patients is effective but may not convey the same long-term benefits as face-to-face therapy (Mohr et al., 2012). When access to a therapist is not possible, a computerized CBT program called Beating the Blues is an option for management of mild to moderate depression (National Institute for Health and Clinical Excellence, 2006). Although it has not been assessed specifically for older adults, the increasing number of computer-savvy seniors makes this option appealing.

Nonspecific factors such as therapist skill and experience and patient motivation and optimism, as well as compatibility of the dyad, may outweigh the value of a specific therapy brand (Scogin et al., 2005). Older adults often possess wisdom and high emotional intelligence and respond well to psychotherapy (Kraus et al., 2007). Limited but nonetheless promising are reports of psychosocial interventions modeled after disease management programs or psychoeducation that are adjuncts to medication management but are not considered psychotherapy (Whitlock et al., 2009). Ultimately, patient preference and the availability of trained therapists may narrow the choice of interventions to a simple few (Wei et al., 2005; Glick, 2004).

The informed practitioner should be able to direct the patient when the evidence suggests that under certain circumstances one intervention may be preferred over another. Similarly, therapists may incorporate techniques from the array of psychotherapeutic approaches for problems that transcend diagnostic categories such as complicated grief, suicidality, executive dysfunction, and relapse prevention. Indeed, innovation in psychotherapy appears to be more a process of hybridization than speciation (Kennedy, 2005). What follows will orient the practitioner to the range of choices and provide practical guidance without pretending to be a manual of psychotherapies.

PRINCIPLES OF PSYCHOTHERAPY IN LATE LIFE

Niederehe (1996) summarizes the principles of therapy with older persons as follows. First, advanced age itself is not an obstacle to therapy, nor does it predict less favorable outcome. Older adults may be more compliant, less prone to attrition, and more positive toward treatment than younger persons. Techniques with demonstrated effectiveness in younger adults can be extended to older adults as well. Problems with health, principally cognitive impairment and physical illness, make the conduct of therapy more difficult and the outcome less certain. Severity of mental illness, presence of a personality disorder, lack of insight ("psychological mindedness"), low expectations for change, and poor quality of relationship with the therapist (mismatch) are also associated with a less successful outcome.

Therapeutic techniques must be tailored to the older person's cognitive capacity, flexibility, and preferences. Ongoing psychotherapy may augment the effects of antidepressants, minimizing recurrence, yet some older adults prefer medication management only. However, when they are queried, combined medication and psychotherapy is the option chosen by most older adults for severe depression (Hanson & Scogin, 2008). Similarly, difficulty with independent travel and limited physical mobility may allow for few or infrequent visits, making psychotherapy too dilute to be effective. Conversely, the geographic concentration of nursing home residents, homebound patients, and occupants of retirement communities may make an out-of-office psychotherapy practice feasible.

Because a family member often brings the older adult to treatment, the role of family should not be underestimated. Family can maintain help regular visits and sustain optimism for psychotherapy, with which their older relative may have little familiarity. Family may also be the sentinels for relapse or flagging enthusiasm for maintenance medication. The primary care provider, home care agency, senior citizen center, church, or synagogue may also play a supportive sentinel role. The therapist may request the older adult's permission to communicate the general treatment plan to these third parties (Milstein et al., 2005) with the assurance that sensitive personal information will not be disclosed.

Most often the older patient will welcome the therapist's communication with family, and they expect communication with the primary care provider. Indeed among primary care providers the most frequent criticism of psychiatrists is lack of communication (Bartle et al., 1995). Collaboration among the patient, professional, and family caregivers is the definition of teamwork.

Although studies of psychosocial treatments in combination with medication are few, when depression is severe, combined therapy is the rule rather than the exception. Given the serious, at times irreversible consequences of relapse for older patients, the capacity of psychotherapy to sustain adherence to medication may be sufficient justification for periodic visits. Therapeutic goals should be identified more broadly than simply the reduction or elimination of symptoms. Improved or repaired social function individually and within the family, greater self-reliance, reduced need for primary care services, better health care planning, and therapeutic compliance are only some of the examples with tangible benefits. An obvious example is psychotherapy and counseling for family caregivers of persons with dementia. Family caregivers provide the overwhelming amount of noninstitutional, informal (unpaid) dementia care. As such they represent a substantial but vulnerable public health resource. They are more burdened by an elevated risk of depression, loss of social ties, and poorer physical health than their non-caregiver counterparts. Any intervention sustaining the quality and extent of their caregiving has obvious social benefits. And the personal satisfaction they take in being productive caregivers, too often ignored, is equally important.

Finally, the scope of need and potential value of psychosocial interventions in late life far exceed the scientific evidence of efficacy. Most of the evidence is generated by academic mental health specialists working with self-selected, fairly independent older adults for whom measures of benefit are narrowly defined in terms of reduced symptom counts on a mental illness metric. Practitioners then generalize the findings to the average patient in the more typical nonacademic setting. An individualized approach, informed by the best available evidence, with clearly defined, realistic goals should be the target of any intervention, more so with psychotherapy for the older adult.

Some patients will feel too old to change or think the therapist too young to help. The potential limitations of both patient and therapist should be acknowledged but with the caveat that failure is certain only when treatment is never engaged. Older persons often feel stigmatized by both the diagnosis of mental illness and any ongoing mental health service. They may associate psychotherapy with insanity, institutionalization, or lasting dependency on the therapist. Education regarding the scientific basis of modern therapy, the goal of greater rather than less autonomy, and the confidential nature of the enterprise should be provided.

All therapies share a set of common general goals. These include establishing a supportive, optimistic relationship, examining distortions in beliefs and perceptions, addressing conflict and ambivalence, repairing interpersonal or intrapsychic deficits, and restructuring defenses. The more specific goal is change in expressed behavior through individualized treatment (Yasavage & Karasu, 1982; Karasu, 1986). Presented below are psychotherapies adapted to older adult needs (see Table 4.1 for a summary). Other psychosocial interventions are described in Chapter 5. In both chapters, the primary focus is functional outcome, which can be seen as a means to an end—restoration of mood and control of counterproductive impulses. Each therapy defines the problem from the patient's perspective and seeks to limit the field of therapeutic play to the pursuit of realistic outcomes. As a result the initial assessment is critical and time consuming. Family members may be involved in the initial session, and in some of the therapies their ongoing involvement is crucial to success. Confidentiality may be of relative rather than absolute importance for most seniors, whose family and other providers may be directly involved in the request for therapy. But permission to communicate should always be requested rather than be presumed. In addition it is important to determine the extent to which patients and family have congruent goals and shared motivations for treatment. Unrealistic or conflicting expectations should be identified and discussed at the outset.

The Initial Psychotherapy Assessment

The diagnostic assessment of depression in late life is covered in Chapter 1. Here we examine the details of assessment for psychotherapy in old age. Effectiveness is the critical component of any treatment plan, but efficiency is becoming ever more important. Unfortunately, older adults require more time and skill from the clinician because of the complexity of their conditions and longer life histories. During the initial assessment the practitioner needs to be active, structured, and alert to the emotional valence of the patient's comments. A missed opportunity to explore a

TABLE 4.1. Psychotherapies for Older Depressed Adults

Therapy	Distinguishing attributes
Brief psychodynamic therapy	Problem focused, transference not examined, identifies conflicts over dependency and independence, intrapsychic locus, insight oriented.
Emotionally supportive therapy	Maintains present level of function or symptom control through the expression of burdensome feelings without examination of the unconscious or search for insight.
Cognitive-behavioral therapy (CBT)	Directive, symptom-focused techniques practiced outside of therapy; counters misperceptions, mistaken beliefs. Helps depressed elders regulate emotion.
Cognitive bibliotherapy	Self-help format using Burns's (1980) *Feeling Good* (1980) as a workbook to identify and challenge maladaptive cognitions; little contact with therapist.
CBT to combat suicidality	Circumstances, thoughts, feelings, images, beliefs leading up to the attempt are addressed, then reprised at end of treatment to assess benefit.
Behavior therapy	Educational; directed at reducing negative and increasing positive experiences.
Behavioral activation	Uses cognitive techniques to reduce avoidance and rumination associated with counterproductive behavior; activates social networks.
Interpersonal psychotherapy (IPT)	Exploratory; present and future rather than past oriented; focused on interpersonal conflict, role changes, and role deficits.
Interpersonal and social rhythm therapy (IRST)	Focus on maintaining regularity of daily routines and managing disruptors of social rhythm to sustain the emotional quality of roles and relationships.
Reminiscence therapy (life review)	Recall of personal success and failure to master one's present and future. Developed for older adults.
Problem-solving therapy (PST)	Focused on change, narrow and pragmatic; solutions elicited from the patient, not offered by the therapist; may compensate for executive dysfunction.

(continued)

TABLE 4.1. *(continued)*

Therapy	Distinguishing attributes
Dialectical behavior therapy (DBT)	Focus on acceptance of that which cannot be changed, nonjudgmental awareness (mindfulness), distress tolerance, impulse control, acting counter to depressive urges.
Bereavement therapy	Restructuring the experience of the lost loved one and restoration of life goals.
Complicated grief therapy	Employs retelling, imaging of the death scene, imaginary conversations with the deceased to decrease disbelief, longing, bitterness, and intrusive preoccupations.

word or phrase charged with feeling can be recaptured once the clinician recognizes the error—for example, "You mentioned something a moment ago I would like to return to." Time allowed for exposition of a sensitive matter can be managed effectively if the initial inquiry is handled deftly: "All your feelings are important, but we also need to reserve time for discussion of what to do." A more focused, directive approach is better suited to the practice style of a primary care provider as well as to the older person's needs. At the end of the more lengthy initial assessment the therapist prepares the patient for briefer, more focused sessions to follow.

A review of the developmental milestones of late life will inform the practitioner of patterns of mastery and defeat as well as resources for change. When the older patient is distressed by growing dependency and burdening of the family, a brief review of the person's experience with his or her own parents will illuminate expectations of care from the family as well as hopes and fears. Self-defeating or problematic reaction patterns may represent behavior learned from a previous generation. Dissatisfaction with attention from adult children may be based, in part, on an inability to accept unanticipated life changes that can come with advanced age. These may include illness or disability in children or grandchildren as well as the mixed lineage and divided loyalties of family members "blended" by separation and divorce across as many as three generations. Asking about the aftermath of a parent's distant death may inform the therapist about the senior who has recently lost a spouse. Responses to retirement and prior episodes of illness and hospitalization may also be informative. Did the person recover fully, or was there a prolonged period of disability or distress? How were these challenges managed? What resources did the older person marshal for support, and what is now available?

Transference: Hidden Meanings Visibly Expressed

Although transference may not be openly addressed in many forms of brief therapy, an awareness of transference and countertransference is important to any therapeutic relationship (Lazarus & Sadavoy, 1996). Transference is defined as the phenomenon whereby unconscious hopes, fears, and attitudes are evoked in the patient by the therapist. Patient reactions emerge in a predetermined way brought about by real-life contingencies within the therapeutic interaction. Processes outside the patient's immediate awareness distort the relationship with the therapist. Transference in late life has its origin in both childhood and prior adult relationships but is provoked by current circumstances. Certain transferences arise more frequently in late life as the older person encounters the loss of goals and ideals, changes in family and intimate relationships, illness, disability, and the approach of death.

Some older patients initially assume the role of mentor or parent seeking to assist the younger therapist rather than settling into the more direct work of treatment. They may disparage the therapist's capacity to assist so senior a citizen. This "reverse transference" (Grotjahn, 1955) may cloak fears of decline, inferiority, and dependence but often yields to a more productive, realistic alliance. Retirees adjusting to the loss of esteem and rewards in the workplace may experience the therapist as an overbearing, rival sibling who is privileged to win at work what the patient is losing at home. The result is an angry, defeated reaction to the therapy as well as the retirement. The therapist, unable to restore the lost self-esteem immediately, may be seen as a withholding or uncaring parent. Alternatively, narcissistic wounds including the loss of physical or verbal prowess, beauty, stature, or financial power may provoke an idealized, magical transference. Older, frail, and dependent persons may unconsciously see themselves as the powerful, admired masters they imagine their therapists to be.

Hiding beneath the idealization is a desperate sense of inadequacy and vulnerability. A seemingly minor disappointment by the therapist or a trivial turn of events beyond the therapist's control may provoke rage, rejection, or exaggerated dependency. With time and effort fantasies of rescue can be replaced by real adaptation. Patients may also develop a spousal transference following bereavement. The absence of an attentive lover and the feared loss of attractiveness contrast starkly with the undivided attention of the empathic therapist. A frankly erotic transference may emerge in which the initially warm rapport decays into bitterness as the unconscious hopes for restored youth and sexuality are frustrated by the therapist.

However irrational and unconscious transference may be, it is provoked by real events, which have real consequences that will erupt into awareness. For example, the person grieving the death of a spouse or reacting to nursing home admission has reason to be sad and angry. Yet it is the intensity with which the patient reacts to the therapist that indicates the reality of transference. Transference is often described as a defense against fears that would be intolerable were they admitted to consciousness. And transference is, technically speaking, a "resistance" to therapy. Yet skilled practitioners recognize transference as a bridge to achieving a more realistic helpful relationship. Whatever form transference takes, it has meaning for patient and practitioner alike. Having appreciated the transference at the outset of any emotionally charged clinical encounter will allow the practitioner to be more efficient, whether the task is psychotherapy, medication management, or surgery.

Countertransference and the Opportunity for Self-Correction

Originally conceived in psychoanalytic metatheory, countertransference is a measurable phenomenon of thoughts and feelings, unconscious and otherwise, evoked in the therapist by the patient. Practitioners predetermine their level of comfort with older patients by the specialty or area of interest they choose. Infrequent contact and lack of training with older adults makes one more vulnerable to countertransference. Rarely is countertransference a problem until treatment reaches a complex or difficult juncture. However, whether their work is mainly or minimally geriatric, practitioners' awareness of countertransference will help them manage the intense feelings that are routinely evoked in elder care. Lack of such awareness leads to practitioner inefficiency and dissatisfaction for the patient and family. Using their Countertransference Questionnaire with 181 experienced therapists, Betan et al. (2005) identified eight countertransference reactions through factor analysis: (1) overwhelmed/ disorganized; (2) helpless/inadequate; (3) positive; (4) special/overinvolved; (5) sexualized; (6) disengaged; (7) parental/protective; and (8) criticized/mistreated. The reactions related more to patient personality than the therapist's orientation, for example, cognitive-behavioral versus psychodynamic. Thus, among experienced therapists from an array of traditions, characteristic countertransference reactions can be identified. However, it is how countertransference is used for the patient's benefit that will distinguish effective work with older adults.

Lazarus and Sadavoy's (1996) review of therapists' unconscious reactions to the older patient reveals several pitfalls that practitioners should recognize. Bringing these automatic, stereotypical reactions into awareness will enhance rather than constrain the therapeutic task. First is the prejudice of ageism, which views seniors as lacking in appeal, productivity, and capacity for change. The older person's declining vigor and approaching mortality overshadow any value, novelty, or reward that the practitioner might find in the encounter. The practitioner's unresolved conflicts over dependency, illness, and death, rage from or fear of parental rejection, or threatened engulfment may also be evoked. Inadvertent avoidance and distancing result, truncating empathy and making the relationship safe but sterile. Practitioners may also idealize their older patients and the relationship to counter latent hostile or sexual feelings toward parents or the threat of abandonment occasioned by the patient's frailty. Patient biopsychosocial problems may then be reduced to biomedical matters. This fosters an authoritarian stance on the part of the therapist that prevents an exploration of more genuine, complex feelings. The unaware practitioner may engage in an ill-considered power struggle with family over control of the patient in a countertransference-driven sibling or Oedipal rivalry. Forgone opportunities to promote other attachments and activities outside the therapy, failure to terminate after treatment goals are clearly attained, and visits or phone calls that are overlong or indulgent are also examples of countertransference phenomena. For better or worse, whether in attachment or separation, relationships between patients and practitioners are freighted with meanings outside of awareness.

EMOTIONALLY SUPPORTIVE PSYCHOTHERAPY

Supportive emotion-focused therapy is process–experiential and seeks to increase the patients' awareness of their internal emotional world (Greenberg, Rice, & Elliot, 1993). The therapist focuses on being empathetically attuned to the patient's emotional state, developing the therapeutic alliance, and facilitating the patient's direct expression of emotional needs and experience. Techniques may be borrowed from Gestalt therapy, such as the empty chair. This involves the patient speaking to the imaginary presence of emotionally significant persons, symbolized by an empty chair. The approach relies on nonspecific aspects of the treatment, including the bond between patient and therapist and the open expression of emotion. The unburdening of troublesome feelings to a receptive, supportive therapist can be as effective as CBT, though less efficient for depression. Mohr et al. (2005) found CBT to be more effective sooner than supportive emotion-focused therapy for depression associated with multiple sclerosis. Yet after a year there were no significant differences between beneficial results of the two therapies. In contrast, supportive therapy may be less beneficial in the context of executive dysfunction (Alexopoulos, Raue, & Areán, 2003). Instructions for brief assessment of executive dysfunction appear in Chapter 2.

BRIEF PSYCHODYNAMIC PSYCHOTHERAPY

Lazarus and Sadavoy (1996) recommend short-term psychodynamic therapy for older persons with adjustment disorders, grief reactions, and recent onset of traumatic stress disorders. For depression in late life there are at least two randomized controlled trials indicating the benefits of brief psychodynamic therapy (Gallagher-Thompson & Steffen, 1994; Thompson, Gallagher, & Breckinridge, 1987). Brief psychodynamic therapy sessions are limited at the outset to 15 visits. This avoids excessive dependency and helps the patient reestablish a positive sense of self-efficacy. The focus is conflict identification, particularly around dependence and autonomy. The therapist will elicit both conscious and unconscious themes including fears that age has made change or adjustment impossible, problems of survivor guilt, and negative attitudes toward the self and aging. Patients can achieve insight and successfully terminate treatment without long-term supportive care.

GENERAL PRINCIPLES OF CBT

CBT seeks to alter thoughts, feelings, and action by focusing on faulty perceptions and habitual behaviors that the individual can learn to change. CBT has been used to treat a range of specific disorders including depression, anxiety, panic, agoraphobia, obsessive–compulsive disorder, and sleep disturbances. The general approach is directive and educational and requires practice and homework. The therapist is active, and the sessions are structured and problem oriented; the present and future are emphasized over the past. The patient is educated to monitor the thoughts (i.e., "cognitions") associated with emotional, symptomatic episodes. The mediating, moderating effects that thoughts have on feelings and behavior are examined. The patient and therapist then question the logic or validity of these thoughts to identify distortions, misperceptions, and misinterpretations. The patient is asked to query the evidence in support of the misperceptions and to identify contrary evidence or alternative explanations. Characteristic biases of fatalism, nihilism, and negativity are identified, and the patient is asked to consider less biased, reality-oriented possibilities. Finally the patient is taught to identify and change dysfunctional patterns of belief that predispose to aversive experiences. CBT appears straightforward but requires skill and experience to serve severely distressed patients.

CBT *with Older Adults*

For CBT to be effective with older adults, Gallagher and Thompson (1982) suggest the following. Patients need orientation to the approach, with the emphasis placed on their active participation in the treatment. This leads to a sense of mastery over stress. New habits need to be learned to overcome difficulties, and this involves the patient's willingness to try out therapeutic directions. Termination is relative rather than absolute. The patient is invited to return to therapy if new problems emerge or old ones recur. This is seen as another opportunity for success rather than failure. When the problems are long-standing or complicated by personality disorder, the number of sessions may need to be extended. Finally, improvement will be more likely if modest goals are set for the older person with limited resources and difficult life circumstances. Even greater activity and flexibility are necessary for patients with cognition impaired by stroke or other medical disorders or sensory impairments (Thompson et al., 1991). Parts of some sessions may be recorded for playback at home. Homework may require written rather than verbal instructions and may need to be reinforced or repeated before proceeding with the next assignment.

CBT FOR LATE-LIFE DEPRESSION

CBT seeks to alleviate dysphoria by attacking what Beck (1976) called a "cognitive triad" of negativism toward the self, the environment, and the future. The triad is sustained by persistent distorted perceptions and beliefs. Depressed persons see themselves as deficient, incapable, unlovable. The present circumstances seem overwhelming and promise only failure. The future is no better and immutable. For many physically ill older adults the future may seem threatening. Yet most seniors manage to maintain their spirits and contribute to the well-being of family and community. In CBT, the therapist helps the patient to examine pointless self-criticism, loss of positive motivation and reward, indecisiveness, guilt, and shame and the tendency to view problems as insurmountable. This means changing erroneous beliefs and bad habits as well as asking the patient to add more pleasurable activities.

The patient is asked to examine behaviors that perpetuate depression, for example, withdrawal from family, friends, and religious or community support institutions. Several behavioral strategies are invoked. Activities leading to a sense of accomplishment and pleasure are scheduled rather than being left to impulse or others' initiative. Progress is measured by keeping count and assessing the emotional effects of the activities. Pleasurable activities that the patient may have abandoned or never considered are included. Assertiveness rather than passivity is encouraged. For example, the older parent who seeks more time with family is asked to take the initiative and be direct—to state a preference rather than waiting to be invited or telling the family what they should have done. Social skills and activities are also emphasized. Bibliotherapy using Burns's *The Feeling Good Handbook* (1989) or Greenberger and Padesky's (1995) *Mind Over Mood*, self-help guides to a better emotional life, may also be assigned to increase benefits but is not as effective without CBT (Floyd et al., 2004). Because anxiety so frequently accompanies depressive disorders, relaxation training and other techniques employed to treat panic disorder may be employed, as shown in Table 4.2.

CBT TO COMBAT SUICIDALITY

When suicidal thoughts are present, the first step is assessment of risk. (See Table 1.3 in Chapter 1 for risk assessment guidelines.) If the risk of suicide is not imminent, CBT adapted to reduce the risk of self-harm is

TABLE 4.2. Cognitive-Behavioral Therapy for Anxiety Disorders: Teaching and Training of Coping Techniques

1. Psychoeducation
   - Panic, anxiety, and agoraphobia are defined, with symptoms shown to be physically harmless and possible to control.
   - Fears of brain tumor, stroke, heart attack, fainting are debunked.
   - Avoidance behavior and anticipatory anxiety are shown to be counterproductive.
   - Written materials are offered or referred to.

2. Cognitive restructuring
   - Demonstration that certain thoughts provoke or accentuate panic and anxiety.
   - Most recent attack of anxiety or panic is reviewed to elicit the associated internal monologue and test reality.
   - Record thoughts to uncover evidence of jumping to conclusions.
   - "Decatastrophize."

3. Respiratory control
   - Recognition of hyperventilation (rapid, shallow breaths with chest muscles).
   - Practice of diaphragmatic breathing (slow, regular abdominal breaths).

4. Relaxation training
   - Practice of progressive muscle relaxation (see Barlow & Craske, 1989).

5. Controlled provocation of anxiety and panic
   - Visualization and imagery exercises for inoculation.
   - Anxiety-provoking situations (from least to greatest) are progressively imagined and described in detail.
   - Coping strategies are subsequently imagined and applied.
   - Exposure.
   - Interoceptive: Hierarchy of fear-provoking sensations (dizziness, palpitations) are described and rehearsed in therapy.
   - Situational: Anxiety-provoking situations (from least to greatest) and coping responses are rehearsed in therapy and enacted outside.

Note. From Kennedy (2000). Copyright 2000 by The Guilford Press. Reprinted by permission.

appropriate. Table 4.3 outlines CBT adapted for suicidality as well as depression. The therapist explores the patient's motives in an effort to reduce hopelessness and to tip the balance toward survival. Reasons for living, such as family, faith, future goals (modest as they may be), and previous demonstrations of resiliency, are made more salient. The effect, over time, of reinforcing positive, rewarding experience and perceptions is to alleviate depression.

TABLE 4.3. Cognitive-Behavioral Therapy for Depression and Suicidality: Teaching and Training of Coping Techniques

1. Psychoeducation

   - Orientation to the approach with the emphasis on recognizing negativity toward the self, the environment, and the future.
   - Learning habits need to be acquired to overcome difficulties accepting therapeutic suggestions.
   - Examination of depression-perpetuating behaviors.
   - Avoidance behavior is shown to be counterproductive.
   - Written materials are offered or referred to.

2. Cognitive restructuring

   - Demonstrate that certain thoughts are self-defeating.
   - Challenge abandonment of previously rewarding activities.
   - Counter reflexively negative thinking.

   Behaviors

   - Schedule rewarding activities rather than leaving their occurrence to chance.
   - Keep count and assess the impact of pleasurable activities.
   - Assertiveness training.

   If suicidal thoughts are present . . .

   - Explore motives and origins of hopelessness.
   - Reinforce reasons for living (family, faith, even modest goals).

   If a suicide attempt has occurred . . .

   - Structured recall of thoughts, images, stressors, and beliefs preceding the attempt.
   - Identify difficulties with problem solving, impulse control, isolation, treatment adherence.
   - Relapse prevention exercise with recall of events prior to the attempt and review of new coping strategies.
   - Additional sessions if coping remains faulty.

Note. Based on Brown et al. (2005).

However, if a suicide attempt has occurred, a more structured approach is warranted (Wenzel, Beck, & Brown, 2008). Suicidal behavior is viewed as a problematic way of coping distinct from the primary mental disorder. And as such the focus on suicidality is an adjunct to the treatment of depression and will require as many as 10 sessions. The intervention model conceptualizes the suicide attempt as emerging from a crisis. Hopelessness and selective attention predispose the person to become fixated on a suicidal scenario in which thoughts of suicide proceed to suicidal intent. At some pivotal point the person can no longer tolerate the scenario, the threshold is passed, and a suicide attempt follows. In a typical scenario an activating event, such as criticism from a family member, provokes anger, then withdrawal and isolation. Intolerable rage and sadness are then followed by the suicide attempt. The sequence proceeds from affect to behavior to automatic thoughts motivating more intense affect and automatic thoughts establishing suicidal intent and then self-destructive behavior. Deficits in problem-solving skills, recurrent or unremitted depression, and developmental factors such as a suicide in the family create vulnerability. Core beliefs ("I'm just no good") amplified by automatic thoughts ("I can't make this go away") lead to a process where attention is fixated on misery and immutability, attended by a loss of capacity to generate or appreciate alternative solutions to suicide.

Over the first three sessions a safety plan is established that includes recognition of warning signs, coping strategies, supportive relationships, and emergency contacts (clinician, crisis hot line, hospital emergency room). Reminiscence about the family of origin as well milestones of adult life is encouraged to give both patient and therapist a feel for how the past might define the future. Events that led up to the suicidal crisis are reviewed to help the patient elicit the preceding cascade of thoughts, feelings, and behaviors. Core beliefs and automatic thoughts emerge, as do vulnerabilities that might be mitigated. By session four behavioral strategies are identified and prioritized for implementation. This will include exploring ways the patient might increase the frequency of pleasurable activities, improve adherence with other interventions, and use indicated social services.

Attention is focused on supportive relationships, including maintaining established relationships and attempting to form new ones, as well as altering counterproductive reactions to the behavior of friends and acquaintances, and use of family support. In addition, the patient is asked to construct a hope chest of survival tools that concretize reasons for living. The items might include a picture of grandchild, letters from a niece, poetry treasured for its personal meaning, or a written prayer, all of which can be the focus of a discussion regarding advantages and disadvantages of living. Flash cards for coping, with predetermined solutions to counter automatic thoughts or feelings, can also be included. For example, the coping card with the automatic thought "I'm just no good, it's useless to try" would include the response "Sure, I'm down on myself now, but it doesn't have to last. I've got good and bad in me just like everyone else. If I give it time the good will come out." But to be effective the content of the coping card must be generated by the patient, not the therapist. The therapist uses the process as an example of how problem-solving skills can be advanced by identifying difficulties and structuring realistic priorities for solutions.

During the last three sessions the therapist will again ask the patient to recall the thoughts, images, stressors, and core beliefs that were activated immediately prior to the suicide attempt. Cognitive-behavioral strategies proposed to counter the maladaptive thoughts and beliefs are reviewed. Changes in problem solving, impulse control, and social isolation and treatment adherence are identified and addressed. Prior to termination the therapist will propose a relapse prevention exercise in which the sequence of events, thoughts, feelings, and activities that immediately preceded the suicidal attempt is imagined. The patient is also asked to respond with current skills not available at the time of the even (e.g., "With what you know now, what would you say to yourself? How would you behave differently?" Also, the patient may be asked to imagine a similar situation in the future and to play out a more adaptive pattern of coping strategies. Having primed the patient to reexperience the circumstances leading to the attempt within the session, the therapist listens for patient responses that indicate a more adaptive, less vulnerable stance. Additional sessions may be offered if significant vulnerabilities persist.

Brown et al. (2005), working with a younger adult sample of recent suicide attempters, most of whom reported multiple suicide attempts and major depression, randomized half to receive 10 sessions of CBT specifically adapted to suicidality and half to case management services with routine care. At the end of 18 months of observation, there was significantly less depression and hopelessness, and fewer suicide attempts, in the intervention compared to the routine care group, although there were no differences in the rate of suicidal ideation. Although proven with a high-risk group of younger persons, Brown et al.'s approach described above provides evidence-based direction for practitioners working with suicidal older adults and their families.

BEHAVIOR THERAPY

Behavior therapy for depression emerged from Lewinsohn's (1975) observation that depressed people pursue fewer pleasant activities. Lack of positive reinforcement leads to a downward spiral in mood, generating a depressive disorder. When habitual, depressed mood and withdrawn behavior become resistant to commonsense advice and require a more systematic intervention. Gallagher-Thompson and Thompson (1995) adapted these insights to the treatment of late-life depression. This purely behavioral approach has several elements. First, didactic education informs patients of the underlying theory of depression and identifies examples of both pleasant and unpleasant behaviors and events in everyday experience. The patient assigns a value to each event to construct a hierarchy of opportunities for change. Second, a plan is constructed that specifies which aversive events can be realistically avoided and which pleasant events can be increased. Patient and therapist agree on how often to avoid an unpleasant event or participate in a pleasant one and the duration of each behavior. The patient keeps a log to document performance. For example, if the pleasant event is walking for exercise with a companion, the patient might agree to walk 20 minutes per day three times per week. Improved mood is not expected at the outset, only a new set of behaviors. Gradual improvement follows as the pleasurable events are increased in time or amount. The patient monitors mood with depression scales or a simple linear scale from 1 (totally depressed) to 10 (totally happy). This converts the patient's subjective experience into a quasi-objective measure. As the patient becomes accustomed to self-monitoring, the array of pleasant and unpleasant events is expanded and the contract advanced. As mood and self-assurance improve, more challenging, complicated tasks are incorporated. Ultimately, the patient, free of depressed mood, can abandon the scheduling and record keeping. The activities themselves provide positive reinforcement. The simple theory, commonsense solution, and straightforward technique lend themselves well to work with older persons (Zarit & Zarit, 2006).

BEHAVIORAL ACTIVATION

Behavioral activation therapy concentrates the behavioral approach described above to counteract patterns of avoidance and withdrawal from interpersonal situations, daily-life routine demands, and distressing thoughts or feelings. Patients are taught that avoidance may minimize short-term distress, but in the long run it promotes difficulty by reducing opportunities to elevate mood (positive reinforcement). It also creates or exacerbates problems as a result of the decreased activity. Behavioral activation is offered as a means of breaking the cycle.

Activities and social contexts that are positively reinforcing and con-sistent with the person's long-term goals are identified and encouraged. Specific tactics include self-monitoring, scheduling and structuring of daily activities, rating the pleasure and sense of accomplishment experi-enced during an engaged activity, exploring alternatives, and using role play to counter perceived behavioral obstacles. In addition to the focus on avoidance behaviors, rumination is targeted to move the patient's attention away from the content of ruminative thoughts toward direct, immediate behavior. Although cognitive therapy elements are central to the approach, it is the emphasis on behavior that is thought to yield results that are as robust (Dimidjian et al., 2006) and enduring (Dobson et al., 2008) as cognitive therapy or antidepressant medication.

INTERPERSONAL PSYCHOTHERAPY

IPT was originally developed for the treatment of depression and sub-sequently modified for older adults (Frank et al., 1993). Practitioners of IPT seek behavioral change in present interpersonal relations, which precedes, then promotes the resolution of intrapsychic conflict. There are four common problem areas related to depression in older adults that IPT addresses. First is unresolved bereavement from loss of a spouse, sib-lings, or adult children. Second are role disputes such as marital conflict or family rivalry or dissension. Third are role transitions such as change from employee to retiree, breadwinner to companion, homemaker to caregiver. Fourth are interpersonal deficits resulting in social isolation or difficulty accepting assistance and support. For example, the patient may complain of loneliness but find it difficult to make new friends or unwittingly drive acquaintances away (Zarit & Zarit, 2006). In this instance an interpersonal inventory would identify deficits in initiating and sustaining relationships as problem areas associated with the symp-toms of loneliness and depression.

IPT elicits thoughts and feelings that cause distress and may be changed by focused review (see Table 4.4). The therapist projects opti-mism and empathy, allowing the patient to express difficulties that may be out of awareness, yet a source of the depressive undercurrent. As in CBT, educating the patient about how interpersonal treatment works is as important as establishing rapport. Although IPT is less directive than cognitive-behavioral or problem-solving therapy, the therapist working with the disabled or frail readily provides advice and information (Miller

TABLE 4.4. Interpersonal Psychotherapy for Late-Life Depression

1. Attributes of the approach
   - The therapist is active, not neutral.
   - The target is behavioral change in present interpersonal relations.
   - The work arena is interpersonal rather than intrapsychic.
   - The focus is on short-term goals and problem resolution, not open ended.

2. Typical problem areas
   - Grief and bereavement (loss of spouse, siblings, adult children).
   - Role disputes (marital conflict, family dissension).
   - Role transitions (breadwinner to companion, homemaker to caregiver).
   - Interpersonal deficits (social isolation).

3. Therapist's adaptations for work with elderly adults
   - More directive: dependency needs addressed practically.
   - More supportive: acceptance is often more realistic than change.
   - More flexible scheduling due to transportation, finances, and health.
   - Existential reality of loss, lifelong pathology, advanced age recognized.
   - Unconscious meaning of the therapeutic relationship not interpreted.

Note. From Kennedy (2000). Copyright 2000 by The Guilford Press. Reprinted by permission.

& Silberman, 1996). With the older patient the therapist is active rather than neutral, issue oriented, solution focused, and pragmatic about what should be done. The focus is on behavior, short-term goals, and problem resolution rather than an open-ended, passive exploration. The impact of past relationships on present problems is acknowledged, but the focus is the present and future.

During the assessment phase the therapist explores important personal relations over the patient's life to identify conflicts and problems. Relationships affected by current or previous episodes of depression will also be examined. The approach is explicitly time limited and not designed to change personality, fixed ideas, or delusional material. During the middle phase the therapist pragmatically approaches the patient's dependency needs and limitations due to loss, lifelong psychopathology, and the unavoidable realities of old age. Goals are kept realistic, attainable, and most often modest. Support and reassurance are offered. The therapist may suggest a role-play exercise to uncover and practice new interpersonal skills and responses. Because the older adult may have limited options for new relationships or social situations, the patient is more often advised to tolerate and accept rather than end long-standing problematic relationships. This does not mean ignoring the problem, but rather addressing other problems where satisfaction is more likely. Neither does it mean tolerating abusive or exploitive relationships where safety is compromised and the intervention of adult protective services may be required.

For seniors with impaired cognition the focus may turn to abilities that remain unimpaired and could be optimized to compensate for lost capacities. Also, the therapist may foster an acceptance of increasing dependency and reliance on others as well as new attachments more congruent with current abilities. The therapist should expect to show greater flexibility toward the length of the sessions and missed appointments due to problems with transportation, health, and finances. The unconscious meaning of the therapeutic relationship is generally not interpreted in IPT. Modest gifts are accepted at termination or holidays with appreciation rather than interpretation. During the termination phase goals achieved are reviewed, plans for the future are examined, and thoughts about ending treatment are discussed.

INTERPERSONAL AND SOCIAL RHYTHM THERAPY

Social rhythm therapy arises from the social zeitgeber hypothesis (Ehlers, Frank, & Kupfer, 1988). *Zeitgebers*, a German word translated as "time givers," or more accurately "time setters," are events that entrain the circadian rhythm or, more poetically, set the biological clock (Grandin, Alloy, & Abramson, 2006). In theory, instability and disruptions in personal relationships and daily routines destabilize circadian rhythms, triggering episodes of affective illness in vulnerable individuals. The hypothesis has appeal, given the cyclical nature of bipolar disorder as well as the sleep–wake disturbances that accompany major depressive disorder.

When combined with IPT, the social rhythm component aims to prevent recurrence of depression by stabilizing (sustaining, restoring) both personal and interpersonal routines. Treatment focuses on the relationship between mood and the quality and regularity of social roles and relationships. The patient is asked initially to complete the Social Rhythm Metric to assess and subsequently reinforce the regularity of daily routines. For 1 week the patient records the time at which 17 activities occur each day. Mealtimes, bedtime, getting up, going to work, and engaging in hobbies or leisure pursuits are assigned a score, with higher values indicating greater regularity. Patient and therapist then work on identifying and managing potential disruptors of the social rhythm. Efforts to resolve current disruptive interpersonal problems and prevent their recurrence are emphasized. Sessions last 45 minutes weekly until remission of the current episode of illness, then every other week for 3 months, then monthly. Persons with bipolar I disorder who improve social rhythm regularity experience a reduced likelihood of recurrence (Frank et al., 2005). The component designed originally for younger persons with bipolar illness but applicable to seniors as well addresses the problem of "grief for the loss of the healthy self." Here the patient is helped to mourn the loss of what life might have been were it not for the disorder. Although designed to lessen recurrence in bipolar illness, social rhythm therapy has particular appeal for older depressed persons whose social roles, routines, and networks have diminished due to retirement, bereavement, illness, or disability.

REMINISCENCE THERAPY (LIFE REVIEW)

Reminiscence therapy, also called life review, is offered to the older person who is struggling with troubling events, loss of independence, and the realization of mortality (Butler, 1963). Called the "frailty identity crisis" by Fillit and Butler (2009), this geriatric syndrome is characterized by physical disorders and deficits along with despair, depression, and a general loss of well-being. As described by Korte et al. (2011), the therapist encourages recall of past personal success, failure, or regret. The goal is to help the person find meaning in the present through partial resolution of conflict within the self or with others (Haight, 1992). "Putting one's house in order" aptly describes the concept, which assumes that plasticity of the self endures into advanced age. As in CBT, homework may be assigned, such as review of memorabilia, photos, and journals. These are often brought to the therapy session. The patient may be asked to write an autobiography or offered the opportunity to reunite with friends or family. In addition to solving old problems, the patient may find an increased tolerance for conflict, a reduction in guilt and fear, enhanced creativity, and a sense of giving and acceptance of life circumstances (Butler & Lewis, 1977).

Scogin et al. (2005) examined five randomized controlled trials in which depressive symptoms were significantly reduced with reminiscence therapy, compared to wait-list or no treatment. Reminiscence therapy was also beneficial for depression, although not as beneficial as problem solving or goal-directed therapy. Bohlmeijer et al. (2007) reviewed 15 controlled-outcome studies of reminiscence and life review. They found an effect size of 0.54, indicating moderate influence on life satisfaction and well-being. Life review was significantly more beneficial than simple reminiscence. Community-residing older adults benefited more than nursing home residents. More recently Korte et al. (2011) randomized 202 older adults 55 years of age and older with mild to moderately severe depressive symptoms to routine care or life review conducted in groups of four to six persons. Those with major depression or suicidal ideas were excluded. The intervention included eight 2-hour sessions of structured life review focused on the integration of past events, their influence, personal values, and self-efficacy. Participants were asked to recall past negative experiences and coping strategies but also to reflect upon positive memories and their meaning in the person's life narrative. They were also encouraged to articulate alternative narratives in which they took responsibility for their choices and then to formulate goals for the future. Compared to those in routine care, persons in the intervention group experienced a significant reduction in depression after 8 weeks, and the improvement endured for 9 months thereafter. Age, gender, education, and concurrent medical conditions did not affect the outcome. However, introverts and those whose only motivation to reminisce was to relieve boredom fared less well.

The technique may be the treatment of choice for those traumatized by overwhelming stress, such as survivors of the European Holocaust. Tauber's (1998) *In the Other Chair* and Novick's (1999) *The Holocaust in American Life* provide historical as well as personal background to inform the therapist. Clearly some persons need to keep old wounds covered (Kahana, Kahana, & Harel, 1988). But more often survivors of trauma are responding to the veiled preferences of others, who would rather not be burdened or who would trivialize the events with superficial identification. Themes of survivor guilt, helpless rage, lasting resentment, alienation ("you can't understand, you weren't there"), entitlement, cynicism, distrust, and the futility of suffering challenge the therapist's endurance. Recollections of betrayal, desecration, humiliation, and incomprehensible loss (e.g., the murder of one's child) may overwhelm the therapist.

However, the therapist's willingness to listen if the patient is willing to talk is a powerful incentive as well as protection against damaging intrusion. Clearly the therapist will never fully realize the patient's experience. However, meaning and understanding are both possible provided the patient is willing to speak and remember. The interchange can be crucial to coping with life-threatening illness, injury, bereavement, or nursing home admission that may evoke memories of catastrophic events. Accepting help during the frail, next-to-last stage of life fosters a "responsible dependency" that promotes autonomy rather than accelerating helplessness (Fillit & Butler, 2009). The benefits of reminiscence therapy suggest that "medically justified" treatment of human suffering transcends diagnostic nomenclature.

But the Holocaust is only one example of a man-made disaster. Increasingly, the public health perspective on large-scale traumatic events is the realization that they cannot be wholly prevented. What can be prevented is lack of preparedness, and the preparedness needs to extend beyond coping with the immediate physical depredations. Sakauye et al. (2009) discuss the aftermath of Hurricane Katrina and how programs for older adults, particularly those who are more vulnerable due to frailty or dementia, must be included in public policies of preparedness, and both early and later response efforts. Sadly, the number of older adults traumatized earlier in life will not approach zero.

PROBLEM-SOLVING THERAPY

PST is collaborative, directive, and brief, usually limited to six sessions. See Table 4.5 for an overview of its main components. Nezu, Nezu, and Perri (1989) identify four goals of PST. The first is improving the patient's awareness that current life problems are directly related to current symptoms. Problems are inevitable, but effective solutions can lessen one's emotional vulnerability. The second goal is to increase the patient's capacity to describe problems such that concrete, realistic solutions emerge. The third is to apply structured problem-solving procedures to current difficulties with the expectation that future obstacles can be problem-solved successfully. The fourth goal is positive experiences with problem solving so that confidence is increased and self-efficacy enhanced.

To begin, written lists are created in the therapy session and homework assigned. The patient, not the therapist, specifies and prioritizes problems, whether they are thoughts, feelings of fatigue, loss of interest, anxiety or depression, or interpersonal difficulties. The patient and therapist together assess circumstances surrounding the problem. The therapist urges the patient to formulate a realistic approach as well as to

TABLE 4.5. Problem-Solving Therapy

1. The target is personal problems, rather than generic skills acquisition.
    - Defining, dissecting the determinants of the problem
    - Setting realistic goals
    - Generating multiple alternative solutions
    - Establishing guidelines for decision making
    - Assessing and choosing the solution
    - Putting the solution in place
    - Success assessment or return to earlier steps

2. "Active ingredients"
    - Behavioral activation
    - Increased exposure to positive experience
    - Enhanced interpersonal sensitivity
    - Remediation of deficits in communication

3. May be used to address executive deficits such as . . .
    - Lack of interest in activities
    - Psychomotor retardation
    - Reduced insight
    - Suspiciousness
    - Behavioral disability

Note. Based on Alexopoulos, Raue, and Areán (2003).

triage problems with less probability of change to a lower priority. Once a problem is identified and its determinants are specified, the patient generates a short list of possible solutions with the assistance of the therapist.

For each solution, advantages and disadvantages are recorded to rank the solutions from most to least difficult to achieve. The patient's pessimism ("It will never work") and lapses in motivation ("I forgot to practice") are addressed by again taking the problem-solving approach. However, the focus is kept purposefully on the initial problem the patient identified to minimize distraction and diffusion of effort. The therapist will also remind the patient that the number of sessions set aside may be specific to the identified problem and that additional problems may be beyond the scope of the present therapy. Clearly, genuine obstacles may arise during therapy and displace the identified problem. Nonetheless, the aim is to keep the patient and therapist focused on one problem at a time when realistic solutions have a high likelihood of success.

In randomized controlled trials of interventions for minor depression or dysthymia in primary care settings, neither PST nor paroxetine were superior to placebo in helping patients achieve remission (Frank et al., 2002). The majority of persons who had received medication or psychotherapy and experienced remission discontinued the intervention at the end of the trial, yet were considered recovered 25 weeks after starting the study (Oxman et al., 2001). However, the response rate among the placebo group was greater than expected. When coupled with the spontaneous remission rates seen in patients with minor depression in primary care, it may well be that the added but nonspecific attention given the placebo group functioned as low-dose therapy. Moreover, because of its brevity and narrow focus, PST shows promise of usefulness in home care settings (Gum & Areán, 2004). Of particular note is the promise of PST for reducing disability among older adults with executive dysfunction. Alexopoulos et al. (2003) found PST superior to supportive therapy in the domains of decision making and generation of alternative solutions to personal problems among persons with major depression complicated by executive dysfunction.

When modified for primary care (PST-PC) populations (Hegel et al., 2004) and integrated into primary care sites by trained therapists (see Table 4.6), it achieved superior depression care outcomes, both symptomatic and functional, compared to generic psychotherapy by community-based providers (Areán et al., 2008a). However, doing so required treatment delivered by therapeutic algorithm to ensure that therapists followed protocol. Integration without guideline-directed therapy may enhance access but not necessarily improve outcomes (Areán et al., 2008b).

DIALECTICAL BEHAVIOR THERAPY

Dialectical behavior therapy (DBT) was originally developed for younger patients with borderline personality disorders, volatile personal relations, and self-destructive impulsiveness, but there are also reports of its use for depression in late life (Lynch et al., 2003). Given its origins, the approach may be particularly worthwhile when depression is complicated by the dramatic, impulse-ridden personality disorders (antisocial, narcissistic, borderline, histrionic). DBT teaches a set of core skills that include "radical acceptance," "mindfulness," "distress tolerance," "opposite action," and increased interpersonal effectiveness, which are defined in operational terms.

In DBT, "dialectical dilemmas" represent extreme poles of emotional, cognitive, and behavioral states. These are countered by the

TABLE 4.6. Problem-Solving Therapy for Primary Care (PST-PC): Seven Steps in Four to Six Sessions

Step 1: Specifying the problem

- Cleary defined and feasible
- Defined in objective rather than subjective terms
- Exploration, clarification of the problem
- Complex problem reduced to component parts

Step 2: Setting realistic goals, realistic solutions

- Objective, behavioral goal
- Defined in behavioral rather than emotional terms
- Goal is feasible, achievable, or needs to be refined
- Goal follows logically from the defined problem

Step 3: Creating several possible solutions

- Brainstorming for multiple choices
- Choices from the patient rather than the therapist
- Suspend judgment; solutions are always "more or less feasible," not "good/bad"

Step 4: Setting up the decision-making process

- Start by eliciting major themes from step 1
- Weigh pros and cons of the solution for self and others
- Compare solutions but keep all choices on the table

Step 5: Making the choice

- The process is systematic and deliberative
- Solutions must meet the stated goals
- Undesirable impact defined and limited

Step 6: Putting the chosen solution in place

- Step-by-step tasks (behaviors) are specified
- Each step is relevant to the solution
- Each behavior must be feasible

Step 7: Reinforcement by outcome evaluation

- Homework tasks and behaviors reviewed
- Failures and successes examined
- Problem-solving approach reinforced
- Schedule of pleasant activities reviewed

Note. Adapted from Hegel et al. (2004). Adapted with permission from the Society of Teachers of Family Medicine, *www.stfm.org.*

introduction of more flexible, balanced adaptive responses. On the one hand, the therapy focuses on acceptance of that which cannot be changed. On the other hand, it focuses on problem solving and change. Acceptance and change are the core dialectic in the therapy. DBT fosters mindful awareness without self-criticism. The patient is asked to adopt a sense of objectivity rather than reflexively assuming that feelings are intolerable or that damaged relationships are beyond salvage. Patients are taught self-monitoring skills to be practiced as part of a daily routine. Distress tolerance is emphasized and augmented by planning how to act counter depressive or self-destructive urges. Personality and coping styles that predispose the person to recurrence of depression are a major concern. These include ambivalence over emotional expression, avoidant coping, excess, and overly sensitive interpersonal reactivity. Patient and therapist work to reduce feelings of being overwhelmed and attain improvement in other areas, including willingness to seek social support, being less likely to take out frustrations on others, feeling greater autonomy during stress, and using planning to cope with stressful events. Patients become less concerned about being liked or worried about hurting others' feelings when they say no to requests. They are also less likely to feel responsible for other people's problems. DBT is outlined in Table 4.7.

In the study by Lynch et al. (2003), depressed adults ages 60 and over participated in 14 skills training group sessions of 2 hours each over 28 weeks. These were augmented with a half-hour weekly telephone coaching session from an individual therapist to reinforce skills maintenance over 28 weeks. The randomized study compared DBT with an antidepressant to an antidepressant only. Patients from both groups exhibited equivalent remission rates during care. However, 6 months following the intervention, 75% of DBT plus medication patients remained in remission compared to 31% of the antidepressant only group. In addition, the DBT group showed significant improvements in independence and adaptive coping. This suggests that targeted vulnerabilities were indeed modified more by the therapy rather than by the antidepressant.

PSYCHOTHERAPY FOR BEREAVEMENT

Bereavement is a major, predictable life event among older adults and a frequent occurrence in geriatric care. With advanced age, fewer of

TABLE 4.7. Dialectical Behavior Therapy

1. Achieving a flexible balance between emotional, cognitive, and behavioral poles, or "dialectical dilemmas"
   - "Radical acceptance"
     o Acceptance of that which cannot be changed
   - "Mindfulness"
     o Self-awareness (observation) without judgmental response
     o Attentional control (priority of focus)
   - "Distress tolerance"
     o Minimizing impulsive responses
   - "Opposite action"
     o Behaving counter to depressive or impulsive urges
   - Increased interpersonal effectiveness

2. Focus on behavior and rigid, maladaptive coping styles
   - Mindfulness training and daily practice
   - Distress tolerance training (impulse control)
     o Suicidal thought
     o Strong negative emotions
     o Distressing memories
     o Stressful situations
   - Emotion regulation skills
     o Identification and labeling of emotions
     o Understand the function of emotions
     o When to accept and when to change an emotion
     o Emotional change strategies
   - Interpersonal effectiveness skills
     o Making requests
     o Accepting help
     o Refusing requests without losing the relationship
     o Reduced interpersonal reactivity (excessive sensitivity)
     o Maintaining a sense of self-respect
   - Problem solving
     o Active rather than avoidant
     o Rational rather than emotional
     o Accepting reality

Note. Based on Lynch et al. (2003).

the senior's friends and siblings remain. Spousal bereavement is more prevalent among older women, whose survival advantage over their husbands is countered by a greater likelihood of disability, solitary living, and nursing home admission. Also, with increasing life spans older adults will more frequently live through the loss of an adult child. The death of a grandchild, particularly in large families, is not entirely remote. Most older persons will not perceive bereavement to be a problem in need professional attention (Shuchter & Zisook, 1993). However, bereavement late in life has a demonstrable impact on mortality. Bereaved older adults are also more likely to develop a major depressive episode within the year after their loss than younger persons. As a result, the practitioner should have the skills for the brief psychological treatment of the bereaved, and also to recognize cases when grief is complicated by a major depressive disorder. This is especially important for the older patient who is of advanced age, lives alone, or has few social contacts.

In my experience, most older bereaved patients are not surprised by the emptiness, sadness, and loneliness, and the preoccupation with their lost loved one. The hallucinated scent, sight, or feel of the deceased spouse, which are common, rarely provoke fears of insanity and may evoke comforting memories. However, the fatigue, anger, irritability, insomnia, and social isolation are unexpected and unwelcome. Ambivalent past relations fraught with unresolved resentments or episodes of abuse may lead to particularly complicated grief reactions. Childless older adults and older men dependent upon their wives for a social life may find the social isolation inescapable. The principles of therapy with the bereaved are straightforward and incorporate cognitive-behavioral and psychodynamic elements. Although they apply to the loss of any family member or intimate friend, the following techniques are applied to spousal bereavement.

For patients seen in referral by a mental health specialist and those for whom several sessions seem indicated, Miller et al. (2001) recommend starting with an interpersonal inventory of the bereaved. To what extent was the deceased responsible for social and financial transactions and who will assist in his or her absence? What practical adjustments must be made to manage without the spouse? Has the survivor independent social or leisure pursuits, or were they shared and dependent upon the deceased? What were the circumstances of death? Was it sudden, expected, or suicidal?

The patient may be asked to bring in old photos of the deceased spouse. These invariably evoke patient memories and spark the therapist's curiosity. To balance more negative feelings, the therapist can ask how the couple first met, what their shared leisure interests and life accomplishments were, and what the deceased's reaction was to the births of their children. Here the purpose is to give the therapist insight into the relationship as well as a more vivid picture of the lost spouse. For the patient, sharing positive memories reinforces the lasting value of the relationship as well as making it more acceptable to express less pleasant recollections. The ultimate goal is to help the bereaved find comfort in the past relationship that will make the future possible to bear. The purpose is not to engender a new dependency but rather to demonstrate that existing relationships can be renewed or expanded. The patient should seek to reestablish life's routine and social rhythm. Regular sleep, exercise, attendance at religious facilities or senior centers, and participation in volunteer organizations and family affairs should be encouraged. The person who complains of being too sad to be with others is certainly too sad to be alone.

When the tears, sleep disturbance, weight loss, and helplessness are severe, persistent, or disabling, medication is indicated. The passive wish for death is not uncommon in bereavement, but intrusive thoughts of suicide or suicidal methods should be taken as signaling major depression. Increased alcohol intake, misuse of analgesics, or neglected life-saving medications (hypoglycemics, antihypertensives, antianginal, antiarrhythmics) approach criteria for major depression and call for a more aggressive intervention. Short-lived sedatives (zolpidem, zaleplon, eszopiclone) or a melatonin receptor agonist (ramelteon) may be of considerable benefit, but a sedative antidepressant (nortriptyline, paroxetine, mirtazapine) is preferred if the symptom profile approaches major depression criteria. Patients requiring a sedative for more than 2 weeks should be evaluated for sleep hygiene counseling or depressive disorder. The bereaved patient's somatic preoccupation or fears of undetected illness do not necessarily indicate the emergence of psychosis. However, undue suspiciousness, refusal of companionship from family or friends, or extreme isolation suggests a paranoid reaction, particularly if frank delusions are in evidence. Without a past history of similar episodes, the correct diagnosis may be brief psychotic reaction, and an antipsychotic should be prescribed with planned withdrawal within the coming months. It is important to recall that sleep deprivation can also precipitate brief psychosis.

PSYCHOTHERAPY FOR COMPLICATED GRIEF

Bereavement is considered "complicated grief" when it evolves into a set of disruptive persistent cognitions and behaviors. As defined in DSM-5, persistent complex bereavement disorder is included in the "Other Specified Trauma- and Stressor-Related Disorders" and is considered different from adjustment disorder due to duration greater than 6 months following the stressful event. More specifically, Shear et al. (2005) characterize complicated grief with five elements: (1) a sense of disbelief regarding the death; (2) anger and bitterness over the loss; (3) recurrent waves of painful yearning for the deceased; (4) preoccupation with the lost loved one; and (5) intrusive thoughts related to the death. Avoidance of an expanding array of situations and activities that remind the person of the loss reinforces the preoccupation and truncates opportunities to recover spontaneously. Moreover, treatments for bereavement-related depression are minimally beneficial for symptoms of complicated grief (Reynolds et al., 1999; Pearlman et al., 2014). Although resembling PTSD, factor analyses demonstrate that the symptoms of complicated grief load separately from both depression and anxiety. Shear et al. (2005) describe a psychotherapy for symptoms of complicated grief that achieved superior results compared to IPT. Although therapy for complicated grief is similar to IPT for the bereaved, it incorporates imaginal and in vivo exposure techniques common to work with patients who have PTSD. Combining psychotherapy for complicated grief with an SSRI promotes greater adherence to the therapy and better overall outcomes and is preferred to psychotherapy alone.

As shown in Table 4.8, the introductory three-session phase of the 15-session program, the therapist provides information to distinguish normal bereavement from complicated grief, including a model of adaptive coping that includes not only adjustment to the loss but also restoration of life's satisfactions. The model portrays optimal bereavement as a process alternating between attention to the loss and restorative behavior and entails a focus on personal life goals. Motivational interviewing techniques are used to establish how life would be different had the loss never occurred and to identify goals. Ultimately the loss is to be integrated into the experience of the bereaved rather than overshadowing it. In the third session the patient is encouraged to bring a friend or family member whose support and assistance can be enlisted to further elements of the treatment. This is particularly important to help the patient when the time comes to confront previously avoided events and activities.

TABLE 4.8. Therapy for Complicated Grief

1. Introductory phase (sessions 1–3)

    • Assess grief symptoms and maladaptive responses
    • Distinguish between bereavement and complicated grief
    • Identify life goals ("If the grief were not so intense . . .")
    • Prepare for confrontation of loss as well as restoration of life's satisfactions
    • Incorporate elements of motivational interviewing

2. Middle phase: Symptom-specific attack (sessions 4–15)

    • Addressing oscillation between confrontation with, and respite from, the loss
    • Desensitizing exercises to reduce avoidance of situations and activities that provoke longing
    • "Revisiting" the death and tape recording the story for playback at home to reduce symptom intensity and promote detachment ("to put the story away")
    • Promoting a renewed sense of connection through imaginary conversations with the deceased (the patient asks and answers)
    • Reminiscence of both positives and negatives
    • Steps toward achieving life goals identified and encouraged
    • Role transitions and interpersonal disputes addressed

3. Termination (beginning in session 12 or 13, completed by session 16)

    • Review of gains and plans for the future
    • Recognition that symptoms may recur but be less intense, persistent, and disabling
    • Reinforcement that transient symptom recurrence is a reminder of past successful coping rather than failure
    • Booster sessions offered should the need arise.

Note. Based on Shear et al. (2005).

In the middle phase, sessions 4–13, each visit begins with a review of the prior week, moves to a discussion or exercise on the loss and its consequences, followed by activities focused on restoration, and ends with plans for the coming week. IPT techniques, including exploration, the examination of interpersonal interactions, and directive coaching, are used to encourage the acceptance of positive and painful memories. The PTSD-like character of complicated grief is addressed with symptom-specific techniques. These include recounting the circumstances of the death and exercises to confront avoided situations. The therapist asks the patient to do a "revisiting exercise" in which the "story" of the death is related with closed eyes. At critical junctures the therapist will ask the patient to gauge the level of distress associated with various elements of the story. The exercise is audio recorded for patient playback between sessions. The experience of listening to themselves recount the event helps patients detach from the intensity of the experience and places them in the role of therapist. The process will also evoke memories not previously expressed that can be examined in the sessions. Immediately after the first recording the patient is encouraged to examine the experience and then "put the story away" for future reference (Shear & Mulhare, 2008). When the patient is able to complete the home playback without being overwhelmed, the home work is complete.

To reduce the distress of yearning and preoccupation with the loss, and to promote a sense of ongoing connection with the deceased, the patient is asked to carry on a mock conversation. The therapist asks the patient to close his or her eyes and begin speaking to the deceased as if the person could hear and respond. The therapist then directs the patient to play the role of the lost loved one and answer over a period of 10–20 minutes. This call-and-response exercise is facilitated by having the patient complete a set of memory questions focused on positive remembrances, but also inviting reminiscence of the negatives as well. For the restorative component, life goals are evoked from the perspective of "What would you want for yourself if the grief were not so intense?" The therapist then works with the patient to identify ways of recognizing progress toward his or her goals. Concrete, behaviorally operationalized plans are discussed, and the therapist encourages the patient to put them into action. As in conventional IPT, role transitions and disputes are also addressed to reengage the patient in rewarding, satisfying relationships.

The termination phase is introduced in session 13 or 14 and expanded upon in sessions 15 and 16. The patient is reminded that intrusive thoughts and pangs of longing may briefly reappear in the future, triggered by anniversaries or intimate situations. However, they will not be so intense, persistent, or disabling. The patient is informed that a transient recurrence of symptoms does not mean failure. Rather the return of symptoms overcome previously only reinforces the value of steps taken to relieve them in the past. And if the recurrence persists, a short course of therapy may be advised. Residual symptoms of depression, anxiety, or sleep disturbance that have not remitted may require additional sessions.

CONCLUSION

Psychotherapeutic interventions from different traditions offer benefits for older persons with depressive disorders, complicated grief, and suicidality. The differing psychotherapies for late-life depression share common elements that are easily adapted across techniques. These include a problem-focused, here-and-now approach with distinct educational and social components. Homework may be assigned, faulty cognition confronted, and interpersonal changes suggested. For mental health specialists accustomed to psychotherapy with younger persons, necessary adjustments in approach include allowances for sensory impairments and cognitive slowing, and identification of improved function as well as symptom reduction as worthwhile goals. Despite advances in pharmacotherapy, familiarity with psychotherapy will remain critical both for primary care and mental health specialists alike. Greater collaboration with the patient's family and other care providers is likewise important. The next chapter reviews other interventions that focus on family and social support.

CHAPTER 5

Other Psychosocial Interventions

This chapter lists additional psychosocial interventions that can be used to combat depression among older persons with a focus on family and social support interventions. The variety of psychotherapeutic and psychosocial interventions far exceeds the scope of the individual practitioner. Yet as systems of care integrate and coordinate providers across clinic, hospital, subacute, long-term, and home care settings, demand for a greater diversity of interventions will emerge. As recommended for psychotherapeutic interventions in Chapter 4, an evidence-based, individualized approach with realistic, clearly stated goals is advisable for the psychosocial interventions outlined in this chapter. Table 5.1 summarizes the interventions reviewed in this chapter.

SOCIAL SUPPORT INTERVENTION

Social support is generally assessed in behavioral, cognitive, or structural components, reflecting such elements as frequency and type of contact, perceived adequacy of support, and symmetry (give equals take) or size of the support network. If social contact alters depression directly, then interventions should improve the type or frequency of contacts. However, a number of studies suggest that it is perceived emotional support that has the more meaningful impact on physical and mental health. If

TABLE 5.1. Other Psychosocial Interventions for Older Depressed Adults

Intervention	Distinguishing attributes
Social support intervention (SSI)	Encourages social outreach, network development; counters thoughts that preempt formation of supportive relationships; enhances social communication and assertiveness skills
Dementia caregiver counseling	Focused on the caregiver role, combines elements of cognitive-behavioral and interpersonal therapy
Control-relevant intervention	Adaptation of behavioral, problem-solving, and social support interventions to provide greater sense of autonomy to depressed nursing home residents
Treatment Initiation Program (TIP)	Early intervention to address the older adult's attitudes about depression and treatment including perceived need for care and stigma of illness and treatment
Family-focused therapy (FFT)	Incorporates psychoeducation with enhancement of communication skills and behaviors, along with relapse prevention planning
Telephone-facilitated care	Facilitates treatment of depression in primary care in a disease management model that encourages adherence without directly providing psychotherapy

social support influences depression through perceived adequacy, then interventions should focus on the patient's perceptions and cognitive process. In contrast, instrumental support for activities of daily living is either unrelated to or negatively associated with well-being (Bolger, Zuckerman, & Kessler, 2000; Lakey & Lutz, 1996; Oxman & Hull, 1997; Wethington & Kessler, 1986).

Oxman et al. (2001) studied treatment response and naturally occurring social support among depressed seniors randomized to paroxetine, PST, or placebo. In the placebo group, persons expressing higher levels of perceived social support experienced decreases in subthreshold depression. Neither of the two active treatment groups exhibited this phenomenon, suggesting the potential value of efforts to change perceived social support in milder depressions. In a longitudinal study of clinically depressed older patients, Bosworth et al. (2002) found that baseline perceived social support was as important as clinical and diagnostic variables in predicting the remission of depressive symptoms.

Given the same level of actual support, some persons will see particular relationships as more or less satisfactory than others (Lakey &
Lutz, 1996). For individuals with low perceived support, techniques from
cognitive therapy (Beck, Kovacs, & Weissman, 1979) offer the means to
address the person's interpretive bias (Lakey & Lutz, 1996). These techniques focus on altering distorted, unrealistic perceptions of individual
supportive relationships. Perceptions of support from specific relationships tend to be distinct from perceptions of support in general (Pierce,
Sarason, & Sarason, 1991; Sarason et al., 1990). And the opportunity
to alter perceptions is greatest when the need for support is expressed
during a crisis (Beach, Fincham, & Katz, 1996).

The Enhancing Recovery in Coronary Heart Disease (ENRICHD)
study employed a systematic psychosocial intervention to increase social
support and alleviate depression in older adults following acute myocardial infarction (ENRICHD Investigators, 2001). The ENRICHD social
support intervention (SSI) utilizes behavioral, cognitive, and social network approaches to enhance perceived emotional support. The intervention is an outgrowth of both CBT (Rush & Beck, 1978) and social-
cognitive theory (Bandura, 1986), in which psychosocial functioning is
seen as emerging from the interplay of cognitive, behavioral, and environmental elements. SSI seeks to highlight the patient's behavioral reper-
toire, cognitive schema, and network interactions, especially those with
family. Indeed, among persons with chronic illness, psychosocial interventions are more likely to have positive effects on depression when they
include family members (Martire et al., 2004).

In practice, SSI aims to socially activate the person through patient
(rather than therapist) problem solving, altering counterproductive automatic thoughts and augmenting coping skills (Berkman et al., 2003).
Table 5.2 summarizes the key features of SSI. A major goal is the alteration of perceived emotional support through modification of environmental, behavioral, and cognitive elements that foster the perception
of inadequate support. Network interactions including marriage and
family are identified to prioritize modifiable factors deemed responsible
for the perception of inadequate support. The intervention is tailored to
the individual's deficits in psychosocial functioning, which are identified using the Social Networks in Adult Life questionnaire. Counseling is then directed at specific problems in social behaviors and beliefs
with one or more work modules. For example, social isolation would be
conceptualized as an environmental deficit requiring the outreach and
network development module. Automatic thoughts that reflexively block

TABLE 5.2. Social Support Intervention

1. Seeks to socially activate the person through . . .
   - Active problem solving.
   - Alteration of counterproductive automatic thoughts.
   - Enhanced coping skills.

2. Alteration of perceived emotional support through . . .
   - Modification of environmental, behavioral, and cognitive impediments.
   - Inclusion of marital, family, and network interactions.
   - Identification of modifiable attributes deemed most responsible for participant's perception of inadequate emotional support.

3. Intervention tailored to the individual's deficits in psychosocial functioning with the Social Networks in Adult Life questionnaire.
   - Counseling mapped onto specific problems
   - Specific problem modules
   - Social isolation, environmental deficit
   - Social outreach and network development modules
   - Automatic thoughts that negate opportunities for supportive relationships
   - Cognitive therapy module
   - Ineffective communication and passivity
   - Social communication and assertiveness modules

4. Involvement of network members is a key component
   - Potential but currently disengaged sources of support are identified
   - Network members are connected to the therapeutic process
   - Focus remains the participant's adjustment

Note. Based on Blumenthal et al. (2003).

opportunities for support would be countered with the cognitive therapy module. Social passivity and ineffective communication patterns would be targeted with the assertiveness and social communication module.

Involvement of network members is a key therapeutic component requiring the identification of potential but currently disengaged sources of emotional support and including them in the therapeutic process. However, when a network member attends the therapy the focus remains the patient's adjustment. Although SSI did not reduce mortality in the ENRICHD study, it was associated with a reduction in depression and improved support. And all study participants received enhanced "routine" care as evidenced by increased access to depression monitoring, antidepressant medications, and psychiatric consultation. Thus the possibility that the supportive nature of study participation was beneficial cannot be excluded. Indeed, patients who received antidepressant medication from their primary care provider or a psychiatrist either before or after randomization to SSI experienced significantly less morbidity and mortality (Taylor et al., 2005).

CHARACTERIZATION OF FAMILY CAREGIVER DEPRESSION AND BURDEN: 1980–2014

The overlapping roles of primary care practitioners and mental health specialists are nowhere more evident than in the needs of dementia caregivers. Family members remain the mainstay of dementia care in the community. Characterization of burden has evolved substantially, leading to an array of effective interventions. Caregiving burden has long been recognized as a major public health concern. Early studies indicated that caregiver burden could be reduced and nursing home admission delayed (Mittelman et al., 1995). With support and training, caregivers could reduce their depressive symptoms and those in their relatives needing care as well (Teri et al., 1997). While considerable attention has been devoted to the distress associated with caring for someone with dementia in the community (Cohen & Eisdorfer, 1988), less has been directed to caregivers once their family member has been admitted to a nursing home. In 1996 Butler already suggested that efforts to contain Medicare and Medicaid expenditures for home care and nursing facilities would threaten to increase the burden expected of family members (Butler, 1996). Their burdens were already substantial. Gallagher and associates found that 46% of caregivers seeking help met diagnostic criteria for depression; even among those not seeking help, 18% met criteria for depression (Gallagher et al., 1989).

Family assistance with activities of daily living may decline after nursing home admission without relieving the caregiver's perceived burden (Light, Niederhe, & Lebowitz, 1994; Zarit & Whitlach, 1992). When compared to caregivers with a cognitively impaired relative in the community, family caregivers of nursing home residents were as distressed as the community group (George, 1994). Indeed, more than 80% of community caregivers do not relinquish the role once their relative is admitted (Kiecolt-Gleser et al., 1991). Although caregivers were accurate in assessing the level of impairment in their relative with dementia (Reifler, Cox, & Hanley, 1981), the severity of impairment does not explain the caregiver's sense of burden or depression (Zarit, Peterson, &

Bach-Peterson, 1980). Caregiver burden is an independent predictor of institutionalization beyond that which might be explained by the relative's cognitive impairment or physical disability (Dillehay & Sanders, 1990).

Conflicts and distorted beliefs over separation–individuation or "letting go" add to the burden of caregiving (Rose & DelMaestro, 1990). Caregiver spouses may become "shadow residents" of the facility (Riddick et al., 1992), averaging more than 20 hours per week at the home (Zarit & Whitlach, 1992). Caregivers have been compared to military wives whose husbands were declared missing in action. Preoccupation with the individual with dementia and confusion as to where that person fits in the family are associated with caregiver depression (Boss et al., 1990).

More recent analyses of caregiver burden confirm the centrality of the subjective, potentially modifiable aspects of the phenomenon. Van der Lee et al. (2014), in an analysis of 56 studies of determinant models of caregiver burden, found behavioral problems of the care recipients were more significant than need for personal care or extent of cognitive impairment in predicting subjective caregiver burden. In addition to patient behavioral problems, caregiver competence, coping, and personality traits, most notably neuroticism, were the most significant determinants of burden, depression, and mental health. Higher sense of self-efficacy and competence was associated with lesser perceived burden and better mental health. Springate and Tremont (2014) examined the factor structure of the widely used Zarit Burden Interview (Zarit et al., 1980) among 206 family caregivers. Caregiver depression and age predicted their estimate of the impact of caregiving upon the caregivers' lives and feelings of guilt. Patient behavioral problems predicted caregiver frustration and embarrassment. The caregivers' level of satisfaction with their relationship with the patient also predicted frustration and embarrassment, as well as impact of caregiving on their lives. In summary, patient behavior and caregiver depression and perceptions rather than patient dependency would seem the logical avenues for intervention.

INTERVENTIONS FOR CAREGIVER BURDEN AND DEPRESSION

Studies of therapeutic interventions regarding separation–individuation (Mittelman et al., 1995) have employed individual counseling and educational support groups to lessen burden and delay nursing home admission. However, these studies have not addressed the broader purposes, outcomes, and positive personal meaning of caregiving (Nolan, Keady, & Grant, 1995). Questions as to the relevance of caregiver burden after nursing home admission remain. Is excessive caregiver burden an indicator of untreated depression? If not, are family support groups in nursing homes sufficient (Toseland et al., 1992) or are psychiatric services necessary? Are there costs saved through family caregiving in the nursing home as well as in the community? Indeed, family involvement in nursing home care has been linked to improved quality of life for the resident with dementia (Lawton, 1994). However, nursing facilities are not staffed to provide mental health services to families whose distress is an obstacle to the residents' well-being (Robinson, 1990). If the expense of long-term care is capped, will the savings be realized through a transfer of costs to the "hidden victims" (Zarit, Orr, & Zarit, 1985) of dementia, the family members? Thus both before and after nursing home admission, family caregivers (and indirectly the care recipients) are likely to benefit from counseling.

The approach developed by Mittelman and colleagues, "enhanced counseling and support" for the spouses of persons with dementia, consists of five to six sessions with four components. Two sessions of individual caregiver counseling are followed by four sessions with family members. Caregivers are urged to join a dementia support group, and they have ongoing access to on-demand telephone counseling. The individual and family counseling sessions occur over 3 months, but the support groups and telephone access continue to be available. The goals are to enhance social support, foster a more benign appraisal of stressors, and reduce depressive symptoms.

Spousal caregivers randomized to receive all four of the components experienced a number of advantages compared to those who received routine care plus initial evaluation and referral to support groups. The caregiver's self-assessed health declined less rapidly, and the effect remained significant after controlling for satisfaction with social support, depressive symptoms, death, or nursing home placement of the person with dementia (Mittelman et al., 2007). The depressive symptoms declined significantly without an increase in caregiver burden. At the time of and after nursing home admission, caregivers receiving the intervention expressed less caregiver burden and depression (Gaugler et al., 2008). The intervention worked equally well when exported to the United Kingdom and Australia and combined with cholinesterase inhibitor therapy for the care recipient with dementia. Caregivers experienced an ongoing significant decline in depressive symptoms over 2 years compared to the routine care groups (Mittelman et al., 2008).

Zarit and Zarit (2006) have developed an assessment and intervention model to reduce caregiver burden and improve caregiver skills. The assessment entails (1) characterization of problems emanating directly from the patient's needs and behaviors; (2) recognition of secondary stressors that add to caregiver burden but are not patient based; (3) estimating the network of support available from family, friends, and formal (purchased) support services; and (4) the presence of depression or an anxiety disorder. After assessment there is a three-part approach to intervention that involves (1) provision of information regarding the disease and course of illness via counseling and education; (2) specific problem solving through family meetings; and (3) support through individual or peer group work.

Semple (1992) suggests there are three typical conflicts that families will experience in dementia care: first, disagreements and uncertainty over the diagnosis and medical treatment; second, conflict over the quantity and quality of care provided; and third, conflict over who should provide care and to what extent it is a shared rather than delegated burden. Some families are vocal and assertive. Problems are routinely surfaced and negotiated to consensus or open impasse. However, other families expect needs to be met as a matter of entitlement rather than negotiated. Their style may require a more uncovering stance in which diagnosis and prognosis are shared via the authority of the practitioner's concern for the patient with dementia. The goal of the family meeting is to make explicit differing views and to gain consensus on interventions when possible.

Some caregivers are reluctant to make their needs known to other family members or to accept assistance from a home care agency. They are afraid of rejection or of admitting inadequacy. They fear loss of control or assume that no other person could provide adequate care or be accepted by the relative with dementia. The loss of privacy and the economic costs when paid companions enter the home are genuine concerns. In each instance, the caregiver should be asked to consider a trial intervention with the caveat that the need for repeated trials or alternative companions is to be expected.

Zarit and Zarit (2006) note that caregivers usually seek help for their relative, not for themselves, so the initial assessment must begin with the identified patient but transition to the caregiver's needs. At times the caregiver comes prepared with extensive experience, background information, and family support. Others will need time to realize their needs and express their preferences. The practitioner should anticipate the right pace of treatment and allow time for assimilation of new information and adjustment to new roles. Obviously, the completed search for reversible causes of dementia and the prescription of agents to enhance cognition should be confirmed. Stresses secondary to the caregiving task need to be identified both to broaden the scope of potential intervention and to realize the limits of the person's circumstances. For example, is dementia caregiving eroding the caregiver's employment or other family roles? Are the caregiver's medical problems being neglected? Can an accumulation of stress be avoided by anticipation and prioritization? Is respite care in the home with another family member or a paid companion an option? Is respite care in a nursing facility financially feasible to allow the caregiver time for a medical procedure or to attend to financial matters away from home. What is the quality and extent of supportive relationships that can substitute for the caregiver or act as a buffer when stress becomes overwhelming? A family genogram with ages and geographic locations may allow both the practitioner and the caregiver to identify untapped resources as well as clarify limits.

Support for the caregiver is integral to each aspect of intervention. Peer support through dementia caregiver groups is available in community settings through contact with the local Alzheimer's association and at some nursing homes. Peer support will lessen the alienation and sense of inadequacy the caregiver feels. Caregiving tips and experience negotiating community agencies (and practitioners) may be shared, as well as means of overcoming barriers, both practical and emotional. Because the task is one of support, relationships that extend beyond the group are encouraged. However, support groups are not available to, nor are they desired by, all caregivers. A support group in which all the caregivers have late-stage relatives will shock the person whose spouse or sibling is in the early stage of illness. And a support group is no substitute for the ongoing care of the primary practitioner or mental health specialist.

Beyond educational counseling, behavioral techniques, and problem solving, individual support for the caregiver should also focus on treatment of depression and anxiety with adequate attention to sleep disturbance and the potential for substance abuse. Medication may be a necessary adjunct to alleviate symptomatic impairment. And on occasion the caregiver's failing cognition will become a focus of attention. Elements of cognitive-behavioral and interpersonal treatment may be included. Certainly in the initial and final phases of dementia, the caregiver is involved in a grief reaction for which elements of bereavement therapy are appropriate (see Chapter 4). However, what is different about treatment of caregivers is the ongoing and progressive nature of the stress. Some will master the task after brief individual intervention. Others will require a more prolonged effort in which family members, community agencies, and other providers will need to be engaged. Some will not be capable of change due to unrecognized mental disorder, substance abuse, lack of familiarity with medical care, or a developmental disorder. Depending on the locale, educated clergy may assist caregivers and can be a source of both therapeutic support and leverage. However, when psychosis, substance abuse, or suicidality is evident, referral to a mental health specialist is indicated.

Although the scientific literature offers good evidence of benefit from specialized interventions for caregivers (Gallagher-Thompson & Coon, 2007), the vast majority will be seen in primary rather than specialty care venues. Data from two studies indicate that primary care physicians and nurses collaborating with patients with dementia and their family members can substantially improve adherence to guideline-directed dementia care (Vickrey et al., 2008) as well as reduce caregiver depression and distress (Callahan et al., 2006). Equally promising is the Maximizing Independence at home (MIND at home) intervention, which identifies unmet needs, including depression, among cognitively impaired patients and their caregivers (Samus et al., 2014). Nonclinical community workers were overseen by geriatric nurses and a psychiatrist to identify unmet needs in patients and family caregivers in their homes. The result was an individualized care plan that may include referral and linkage to services, provision of dementia education and strategies to build caregiving skills, and care monitoring. After 18 months of observation, intervention participants were less likely to have left home due to either death or institutionalization. They also reported higher quality of life and had significantly fewer unmet needs for safety and advance care planning. However, although this study incorporated the caregiver, its focus was not specifically caregiver burden. Nonetheless, the improved quality of life reported by the patients suggests benefits for caregivers as well.

In summary, an individualized, structured approach to the caregiver will reduce depression and may delay nursing home placement for the person receiving the care. The interventions need not be extensive and do not increase caregiver burden. Many caregivers will cope with a minimum of support and information and can be well served with defined primary care protocols. Others will need referral to community agencies and peer support groups. However, a minority, which will grow in size as the prevalence of dementia increases, will require the assistance of a mental health specialist.

CONTROL-RELEVANT INTERVENTION FOR DEPRESSION IN THE NURSING HOME

Several investigators (Schulz, 1976; Rodin & Langer, 1977) have noted that nursing home residents who are offered greater opportunities to control their daily routine display improved affect. Rosen et al. (1997) randomized 31 cognitively capable nursing home residents with major or minor depression to 6 weeks of control-relevant intervention or care as usual. Those in the intervention group were helped to develop an individualized socialization plan based on personal interests and opportunities to control the timing and content of activities. The intervention included elements of behavioral, problem-solving, and social support therapy but was adapted to the constraints of nursing home life. Personally relevant leisure pursuits or spiritual activities chosen by the resident were identified and coordinated with family visits or facility-based activities. For example, rather than waiting passively for family to visit, the resident was encouraged to schedule a regular, appointed time and to focus the visit on a pleasurable activity such as music or reminiscence of positive memories. The scheduled visits relieved the family of guilt and the resident of uncertainty while focusing on pleasurable activities rather than the unpleasant reality of dependency and confinement. The intervention offered a restored sense of autonomy and predictability for residents and their families and enhanced self-efficacy for staff. Residents who had identified the environment as inadequate to their needs prior to the intervention subsequently experienced significant reductions in depression (Rosen et al., 1997).

THE TREATMENT INITIATION PROGRAM

The Treatment Initiation Program (TIP) is an adjunct for antidepressant pharmacotherapy among older adults with major depression. It includes three 30-minute sessions during the first 6 weeks of medication therapy followed by two follow-up telephone calls 8–10 weeks after initiation. In the first session typical barriers to care are identified. These include (1) misunderstandings about depression and its treatment; (2) perceived need for care; (3) fears of stigma and shame regarding mental illness and therapy; (4) distorted beliefs and thinking patterns associated with depression; and (5) logistical barriers such as transportation, costs of medication, and contact with the prescribing physician. Having identified specific barriers, the therapist is able to individualize the approach. The therapist then uses psychoeducation, cognitive-behavioral and empathic–supportive techniques to reduce obstacles, reduce passivity, and achieve a greater sense of self-efficacy among patients. In a randomized study of older adults treated for depression in a geriatric psychiatry clinic, those receiving TIP exhibited less severity of depression and less hopelessness, and were more likely to remain in treatment 12 and 24 weeks after the initiation of antidepressant therapy (Sirey, Bruce, & Alexopoulos, 2005a). This was despite a lack of difference between the routine care and TIP groups on the number of clinic visits and provision of supportive psychotherapy by clinic social workers.

FAMILY-FOCUSED TREATMENT
FOR BIPOLAR DEPRESSION

Psychosocial interventions for bipolar depression have grown in number and sophistication. Although the efficacy data are based mainly on experience with younger adults, the techniques, with modification, have obvious appeal for older persons and their families hoping to prevent recurrence. Miklowitz and associates (2003) describe a family-focused therapy (FFT) for patients with bipolar disorder and their families that achieves superior medication adherence and reduced hospital readmission rates compared to crisis management or intensive individual therapy alone (see Table 5.3). In addition to a reduction in the risk of hospitalization associated with recurrence (Miklowitz et al., 2007a), improvements in functional outcomes are also observed (Miklowitz et al., 2007b). In accordance with the Systematic Treatment Enhancement Program for Bipolar Disorders (STEP-BD), patients were randomized to collaborative (enhanced) care or to one of three brief but intensive psychosocial interventions. Persons in the collaborative care condition viewed an educational videotape, received a self-care workbook, and were counseled on sleep monitoring and relapse prevention over three 30-minute sessions. The intensive psychosocial interventions applied in three 30-minute sessions included CBT, interpersonal and social rhythm therapy (ISRT), and FFT.

In individual CBT, patients and therapists discussed behavioral activation exercises, problem solving, and cognitive restructuring to

TABLE 5.3. Family-Focused Therapy for Relapse Prevention

1. Psychoeducation
   - Collaboration between patient and family reinforces rather than sacrifices autonomy by preserving independence.
   - Depressed mood (and mania) is part of the illness, not a weakness or moral flaw.
   - Lack of social stimulation, rewarding activities, exercise, and a regular sleep schedule and use of alcohol promote relapse.
   - Medication, psychotherapy, and social support prevent relapse.
   - Psychotherapy counters self-defeating thoughts and perceptions.

2. Training to enhance communication
   - Active listening that seeks clarification rather than closure.
   - Focused rather than global positive and negative feedback.
   - Requests for change framed in the positive rather than the negative.
   - Role-playing assignments.

3. Relapse prevention planning
   - Practice brainstorming to solve the problem of symptom emergence
   - Solutions are selected by the patient and family, with feedback from the therapist
   - Devise and rehearse a relapse prevention drill with a family-wide response plan
   - Risk reduction plan for suicidal ideation
   - Actions family and social supports should institute
   - Threshold for emergency communication/intervention
   - List emergency contact information and backup when one or another professional is not available (physician, therapist, emergency room, 911)

Note. Based on Miklowitz et al. (2003).

reverse negative self-attributions and increase rewarding activities. In ISRT, they explored interpersonal problems and difficulties maintaining a physiologically stable schedule of sleep, waking, and activity to prevent destabilizing social and interpersonal events. For persons with at least one willing family member, FFT focused on shared relapse prevention planning, improved listening and communication, and problem-solving skills. Compared to three sessions of collaborative care, the benefits in relationships and life satisfaction associated with the psychosocial interventions exceeded those expected from improvements in mood. Thus the benefits were not simply attributable to improvements in mood alone. However, for older adults enthusiasm for these psychosocial interventions must be tempered by the frequency with which cognitive impairment accompanies bipolar disorder even when patients are euthymic

(Murphy et al., 1999; Gildengers et al., 2007). For the older patient more exacting cognitive assessment and remediation may be necessary to maximize improvement in function, social roles, and recreational activities (Miklowitz et al., 2007b).

Because FFT involves the patient, family, and practitioner in a collaborative effort to prevent relapse, it is also appealing for recurrent depression, particularly when delusions or suicidality have complicated the illness. At the outset the therapist emphasizes that collaboration between patient and family enhances rather than sacrifices autonomy by preserving independence. A didactic approach is used to reduce shame and stigma by educating the patient and family so they understand that depression and mania are illnesses, not signs of moral weakness. It is the illness that needs to be controlled, not the person. The therapist emphasizes the importance of social stimulation, rewarding activities, physical activity, and a regular sleep–wake schedule, as well as medication, psychotherapy, and social support. The therapist will also conduct training sessions to facilitate communication between the patient and family members. These will include (1) "active listening" that promotes clarification rather than closure; (2) providing specific behaviorally focused, rather than global, positive and negative feedback; (3) framing requests for change in positive, rewarding rather than negative, threatening language; and (4) role-play assignments in which the patient plays the part of a concerned family member and a family member plays the patient.

A significant amount of time is devoted to planning for relapse prevention. As with PST, there is in-session brainstorming on how to react to symptoms should they reemerge. The therapist offers encouragement and feedback about feasibility but ensures that solutions are selected by the patient and family. The therapist may suggest scripting and rehearsing a relapse prevention drill with a family-wide response plan. The plan specifies (1) a risk reduction protocol for suicidal ideation if present; (2) actions family and social supports should take for other emerging symptoms or lapses in medication adherence; (3) a defined threshold for emergency communication and intervention with an advance directive to waive confidentiality; and (4) copies of emergency contact and backup information should one or another professional not be available (physician, therapist, emergency room, 911). The goal is the preservation of independence, conceived as a multilateral effort with responses to specified threats predetermined by patient and family through the help of the therapist. The patient's risk cannot be eliminated, but it can be reduced by procedures that lessen vulnerability and offer both hope and allies.

TELEPHONE-FACILITATED DEPRESSION CARE

Telephone disease management (TDM) of depression (Oslin et al., 2003) was originally developed for the U.S. Department of Veterans Affairs outpatient programs as a Behavioral Health Laboratory (BHL) to reduce depression and at-risk drinking (Zanjani et al., 2008). The BHL is a clinical service designed to help manage the behavioral health needs of veterans seen in primary care. The core assessment of the BHL is a brief structured telephone interview that provides primary care clinicians with a comprehensive assessment of patients' mental health and substance abuse (MH/SA) symptoms. The BHL also offers the option of structured follow-up telephone assessments and serves as a platform for specific disease management programs. The program also incorporates decision support, including triage to specialty MH/SA services. Within the Department of Veterans Affairs, the BHL has been recognized as a "best practice" for identification of and early intervention for MH/SA symptoms in primary care patients. Although the majority of interactions between BHL patients and staff occur by phone, a complex infrastructure supported by an electronic medical record integrates the care protocols across the full chain of care. Evidence suggests that less elaborately networked telephone psychosocial interventions may also be effective for depression.

Mohr et al. (2005) described a 16-week trial comparing telephone-administered CBT to telephone-administered supportive emotion-focused therapy for multiple sclerosis patients suffering a major depressive episode or dysthymia. Both interventions were provided by doctoral-level psychologists following treatment manuals. Half the patients in each group were taking an antidepressant at the outset. Both treatments were effective at 12 months, but CBT achieved superior results at 16 weeks on measures of mood and remission of major depressive disorder. Fewer than 6% across the sample withdrew from the study. Although the mean age was 47 years, the disability associated with multiple sclerosis makes the study informative for older adults, whose depression most often complicates physical conditions. The low attrition rate and more rapid onset of action with CBT suggested that telephone intervention may be a promising alternative when face-to-face therapy is not feasible.

Telephone-facilitated depression care by nonspecialists not located in primary care may be an effective alternative to models that integrate a mental health specialist into the primary care site (Hunkeler et al., 2000; Datto et al., 2003; Oslin et al., 2003; Katon et al., 2000; Unützer et al.,

2002). Facilitators are typically master's-level social workers, psychologists, or registered nurses. Depression care facilitation added to existing disease management programs for diabetes, congestive heart failure, and other chronic conditions in which depression is prevalent (Kennedy & Marcus, 2005) is particularly appealing but remains unproven. The apathy, difficulty concentrating, and executive dysfunction that accompany depression make these patients more likely to experience difficulty adhering to a therapeutic regimen and place them at increased risk for readmission to the hospital (Cooney et al., 2004; Pugh et al., 2003; Alexopoulos et al., 2003). Facilitated care by telephone requires a variety of interactions from the facilitator (Oxman, 2003). These include (1) solving problems caused by barriers such as reluctance to initiate prescribed antidepressant therapy or to communicate difficulties with side effects to the primary care clinician; (2) providing positive reinforcement and praise once barriers are overcome; and (3) monitoring progress, assessing response to treatment, and countering premature discontinuation of medication. The facilitator does not diagnose depression, provide psychotherapy, or indicate a choice of antidepressants, and as such functions more as a technician than a clinician. As a result it may be necessary for a psychiatrist or other mental health professional to contact the primary care provider to initiate antidepressant therapy (Pickett et al., 2014b).

Several studies indicate that depression screening and assessment by phone is valid and reliable. The nine-item Patient Health Questionnaire (PHQ-9; Spitzer, Kroenke, & Williams, 1999), described in Chapter 1 and shown in Table 1.1, is a depression-specific assessment derived from the PRIME-MD, which has been validated for administration by a mental health specialist via a telephone interview (Spitzer et al., 1995). PRIME-MD has been adapted for computer-assisted telephone interviewing in population-based studies (Kobak et al., 1997). Telephone assessments of depressive symptoms using the Center for Epidemiologic Studies Depression Scale compare favorably to in-person assessments (Aneshensel et al., 1982) with no significant differences in item nonresponse, reliability, mean level of depression, or proportion classified as depressed. Furthermore, there were no significant interactions with sociodemographic characteristics between the interview methods. Telephone assessment for depression may be experienced as less intrusive by the patient (Allen et al., 2003).

Telephone screening should include a query for suicidality because persons with suicidal ideation, despite less severe depression, respond better to facilitated than routine care (Bruce et al., 2004). Telephone facilitators need a clear protocol to manage suicide risk. Risk of suicide can be assessed in three steps (Oxman, 2003). First, persons are asked, "Have you had any thoughts that you would be better off dead or of hurting yourself in some way?" Those with any positive response to the question are subsequently asked, "In the last 2 weeks, have you had any thoughts of hurting yourself in some way?" This helps to distinguish active from passive thoughts of death. Those answering no are considered low risk. Those with active thoughts of death are then asked about methods of self harm, plans for suicide, past attempts, and capacity to resist the impulse before the next visit to the primary care provider. Persons answering yes to the possibility of hurting themselves before their next provider visit are considered emergent/high risk and require emergency evaluation through contact with their primary care clinician, emergency room, or 911.

Persons who deny any risk of hurting themselves prior to their next visit but who answer any of the other suicide questions positively are considered to be at urgent/moderate-to-high risk. Persons at urgent risk should be evaluated within 48 hours. In either emergent or urgent risk conditions, the primary care clinician or on-call covering professional should be contacted. If not readily available, a psychiatrist should be reached. For persons at low risk, the primary care clinician is simply informed via routine communication. However, when the facilitator has minimal clinical training, any expression of suicidal ideation should trigger a risk assessment by a mental health specialist.

CONCLUSION

In addition to the psychotherapeutic interventions reviewed in Chapter 4, older depressed adults can benefit from other social and family-focused supportive interventions. Interventions such as the TIP and telephone-facilitated care can enhance the effects of pharmacotherapy. It would be unrealistic to suggest that providers incorporate all these interventions into their practices. But as health care becomes based more on an integrated model of services rather than the individual practitioner, the therapeutic components described above will likely be in demand.

CHAPTER 6

Diet, Supplements, and Exercise

D iet and exercise have long been the cornerstones of good health. Although many practitioners are pessimistic about counseling fewer calories and more activity, the science supporting the benefits of diet and exercise increasingly points to a more palatable, less exhausting approach to achieving healthful goals. Diet and exercise can alter age-related transitional states that lead to disease, so dependency due to illness in old age can be reduced (Hamerman, 2010). Similarly, promoting function is one of the most important means of increasing the chances of remission and recovery from depression. Depressed patients often welcome advice on diet and exercise because it promotes a sense of self-efficacy. Simple suggestions about where to start and why should be part of the behavioral activation routine when beginning any intervention to combat depression. This chapter presents the theory and empirical evidence supporting the role of diet and exercise in combating depression. Although a structured program of physical activity is best, simply providing advice on diet and exercise has measureable benefits (Umpierre et al., 2011).

EVIDENCE LINKING ADVANCED AGE, DIET, AND DEPRESSION

Table 6.1 displays age-related changes in function that lead to decrements in nutrient intake and processing as well as alterations in body

TABLE 6.1. Modifiable Age-Related Functional Changes and Transitions Associated with Disease and Disability

Age-related change in function	Transitional state	Disease or condition leading to disability
↓ Food intake, smell, and taste	Deficits in protein, vitamin D, calcium	Osteomalacia
↓ Bone density	Osteopenia, osteoporosis	Fractures
↓ Muscle mass	Sarcopenia, weakness	Falls
↑ Visceral fat	Increase in inflammatory mediators	Metabolic syndrome of hypertension, hyperglycemia, hyperlipidemia

Note. Adapted from Hamerman (2010). Adapted with permission from the American Geriatrics Society.

composition. These, in turn, predispose one to disease or disability. They include declining food intake related to declines in physical activity and reduced caloric needs. Gustatory and olfactory sensitivity are also reduced, and salt and sweeteners are increased to compensate for loss of flavor. With advanced age there is also an accelerated loss of bone and muscle, and an increase in visceral fat. As they progress, these changes lead to pathological transitional states that are disabling but modifiable with diet and exercise. In addition, dietary patterns associated with depressive disorders elevate the risk of diabetes, cardiovascular disease, and stroke, and are obvious targets for intervention.

Less obvious but perhaps more direct are the pro-inflammatory cytokines, such as interleukins 1 and 6, which are associated with obesity and the metabolic syndrome. As described in Chapter 2, pro-inflammatory cytokines that emanate from adipose tissues elevate glucocorticoids and depress neurogenesis and the production of neurotrophins (Song & Wang, 2010). The loss of neurogenesis and dysregulation of the neurotrophic system are posited to underlie the pathogenesis of depression. And in animal models of depression, these losses can be restored with antidepressants or omega-3 fatty acids.

The most compelling evidence of nutrition's capacity to prevent disease and extend the lifespan comes from calorie restriction studies of laboratory animals. Calorie restriction augments DNA repair, regulates insulin dynamics, reduces oxidative stress, and preserves immune function. Rats whose caloric intake is reduced to near starvation levels experience a 40% increase in lifespan. However, at that level of restriction they cannot reproduce. Ongoing studies of primates offer a less stark comparison. Monkeys whose caloric intake is restricted to 70% of ad libitum fed control animals keep their body weight at young adult levels. The calorie-restricted animals also receive vitamin and mineral supplements. They exhibit lower blood pressure and serum lipids, greater insulin sensitivity, and less diabetes. Less spinal arthritis and cancer are also observed. Illnesses that are often associated with depression in humans are delayed if not prevented. Although the restricted animals are obviously hungry, they are no more aggressive and no less energetic than the ad-libitum-fed group (Colman et al., 2009).

Thus, both advanced age and common physical illnesses can predispose a person to depression through indirect effects of disease and disability but also through the direct impact of cytokines and neurotrophic factors on the brain. Both mechanisms can be altered with diet and exercise.

Is There an Antidepressant Diet?

Adherence to a Mediterranean dietary pattern is thought to reduce the metabolic, inflammatory, and vascular processes involved in the risk of depressive disorders. Rather than restricting calories and fats, the Mediterranean diet is patterned on enhancing the quality of calories and fats. Highly processed foods rich in carbohydrates, which lead to a rapid rise in blood sugar, are replaced by vegetables, fruits, nuts, whole-grain cereals, and legumes. The result is a more nutrient-dense and fiber-enriched meal with a lesser peak in serum glucose and longer-lasting satiety. Ingestion of red meats and whole-fat dairy products high in saturated fats is minimized by the substitution of fish and olive oil creating a more favorable monounsaturated- to saturated-fatty-acid ratio. Moderate alcohol consumption is allowed, generally as red wine. Go to *www.mayoclinic.com/health/mediterranean-diet/CL00011* for detailed advice on food selection and substitution for the Mediterranean diet.

In addition to better glucose metabolism, the Mediterranean diet is associated with lowered blood pressure, less abdominal obesity, and reduced prevalence of the metabolic syndrome, as well as better high-density cholesterol levels. It is also associated with less cardiovascular disease and diabetes, potentially through the preservation of vascular endothelial integrity. Endothelial cells secrete brain-derived neurotrophic factor (BDNF), which promotes neuronal survival and synaptic plasticity and is reduced in depression. Similar to the effect of antidepressants, the Mediterranean diet may support the production of BDNF. Moreover, it substitutes foodstuffs higher in folic acid, B vitamins, and omega-3 fatty acids, all of which are critical to monoamine synthesis and the availability of dopamine, norepinephrine, and serotonin. The simplicity of the diet as well as its theoretical underpinnings make it an appealing addition to the therapeutic regimen for depressed older adults. Empirical evidence suggests it may have a protective effect against incidence or recurrence of depression as well.

Sánchez-Villegas et al. (2009) found an inverse dose–response relationship between levels of adherence to the Mediterranean diet and the risk of receiving a depressive disorder diagnosis or antidepressant medication. Among more than 10,000 university graduates and registered professionals followed for a median of 4.4 years, the hazard ratio for the incidence of depressive disorders was reduced by 25–50% for the four quintiles reporting higher adherence to a Mediterranean pattern of diet. Cox proportionate hazards models were used to adjust for the effects of age, gender, physical activity, total caloric intake, body mass index, and employment status. Participants with cardiovascular disease at baseline were excluded from the analyses. Those with hypertension at the outset or who subsequently developed cardiovascular disease were included. The contributions of prevalent hypertension and incident cardiovascular disease were also controlled. The crude rate for depression in the quintile least adherent to a Mediterranean pattern was 14 depressed persons per 1,000 per year. The crude rates for the upper four quintiles ranged from 8 to 10 cases of depression per 1,000. The favorable hazard ratio for those more adherent could not be explained on the basis of lower body mass index, more activity, fewer calories, younger age, or freedom from cardiovascular disease.

The sample was younger to middle-aged, well-educated residents of Spain, where a Mediterranean diet is common and depressive disorders less prevalent than in Northern Europe. Thus the results may be less informative for older adult primary care patients in the United States and those with a preexisting diagnosis of depression. Clearly, these findings need to be demonstrated in an older clinical sample to be compelling. Nonetheless, the healthy, educated, and Spanish character of the sample makes the detection of a direct protective effect associated with diet noteworthy. For patients and practitioners interested in a diet to combat depression, these data are the best at hand.

VITAMINS, MINERALS, AND SUPPLEMENTS

A number of studies have sought to examine relative vitamin deficiency states as direct contributors to depressive illnesses. Of particular interest have been folate and vitamins B_6 and B_{12}, vitamin D, calcium, omega-3 fatty acids, St. John's wort, and SAM-e. Findings from the scientific literature are reviewed below.

Folate and the B Vitamins

Because folic acid and the B-complex vitamins are involved in the synthesis of serotonin, dopamine, and norepinephrine, there has been considerable interest in their capacity to ameliorate mood disorders. Skarupski et al. (2010) found a lower incidence of depressive symptoms in association with higher intake, including supplementation, of vitamins B_6, B_{12}, and folate among a population of more than 3,000 older community residents. Sachdev et al. (2005) found low folic acid and high homocysteine, but not low vitamin B_{12} levels, were associated with depressive symptoms among community residents ages 60–64. Walker et al. (2010) failed to observe any benefit from folic acid and vitamin B_{12} against depressive symptoms in community residents ages 60–74. Buhr and Bales (2010) describe encouraging findings from their review of the effects of nutritional supplements including folic acid and vitamins B_6 and B_{12}. The American Psychiatric Association Task Force on Complementary and Alternative Medicine concluded that folic acid augmentation of antidepressant treatment is a low-risk and reasonable part of a treatment plan for major depressive disorders. However, the dose and role of folate-related compounds is far from established (Freeman et al., 2010). The B-VITAGE trial (Ford et al., 2010), under way at the time of this writing, will include 300 depressed older adults whose citalopram treatment will be augmented with either placebo or vitamins B_{12} (0.4 mg), B_6 (25 mg), and folic acid (2 mg).

Vitamin D

The need to supplement the diets of older persons with vitamin D is well accepted. The body generates vitamin D in response to sun exposure of the arms and trunk. However, naturally occurring vitamin D levels plunge during winter, especially in the northern latitudes and among persons not exposed to sunlight at other times of year. May et al. (2010) found elevations in depressive symptoms among more than 7,000 cardio-vascular patients ages 50 and over related to vitamin D levels below an estimated optimum of 50 ng/ml. Jorde et al. (2008) found high doses of vitamin D (20,000–40,000 IU per week) ameliorated depressive symptoms in overweight and obese outpatients. A 2010 international panel of experts recommended supplementation with 800 IU 25-hydroxyvitamin D for older adults and institutionalized persons without baseline testing. However, assays of both 25(OH)D(2) and 25(OH)D(3) should be obtained 3 months after beginning supplementation to ensure that a target range of 30 to 40 ng/ml has been attained (Souberbielle et al., 2010). Thus, for depressed older adults a minimum supplementation of 800 IU of colecalciferol 25(OH)D(3) daily seems prudent, but may not be optimal. Bischoff-Ferrari (2009) suggests up to 2,000 IU to achieve optimal serum levels of D_3. However, Li et al. (2013) found insufficient evidence from randomized controlled trials to support the use of vitamin D supplementation specifically to counter depression.

Calcium

Compared to vitamin D, the benefits of added calcium for depression are less certain, although a number of studies have used supplements of both to reduce the risk of osteoporosis and fracture. The Women's Health Initiative (Jackson et al., 2006) found increases in bone density but no significant reduction in the risk of fracture among healthy postmenopausal women given supplements of 1,000 mg calcium as calcium carbonate and 400 IU vitamin D daily. However, the risk of kidney stones was increased. And at least one meta-analysis found a slight increased risk of myocardial infarction when calcium is supplemented without added vitamin D (Bolland et al., 2010).

Nonetheless, there are arguments for recommending calcium supplementation for older depressed patients. First, adequate intake of calcium (1,200 mg daily) and vitamin D along with weight-bearing exercise are recommended to combat the progression of osteoarthritis and associated disability (Buhr & Bales, 2009). Clinical depression may be associated with low bone mass (Rosen, 2009). Second, the use of SSRI depressants may be associated with increased bone loss among depressed persons compared to the older tricyclic antidepressants (Haney & Warden, 2008).

The older person whose activity level and diet are likely to have been degraded by a depressive episode may well need combined vitamin D and calcium supplementation.

Omega-3 Fatty Acids

Eicosapentaenoic acid (EPA) and docosahexaenoic acid (DHA) are polyunsaturated omega-3 fatty acids with proven benefits for health. Omega-3 fatty acids are found in fish and marine sources but are relatively deficient in the American diet. The health benefits are primarily cardiovascular and include reduction of triglyceride levels in hypertriglyceridemia, decreased atherosclerosis, decreased risk of thrombosis and arrhythmias, reduced inflammation, and modest improvement in hypertension. Epidemiological studies have demonstrated an inverse relationship between per capita fish intake and prevalence rates of major depression, postpartum depression, and bipolar disorder. Supplementation with omega-3 fatty acids specifically for depression has shown promise in younger patients (Rocha Araujo, Vilarim, & Nardi, 2010) and older ones as well (Rondanelli et al., 2010). Having reviewed the available evidence, the American Psychiatric Association Task Force on Complementary and Alternative Medicine found "the established general health benefits of omega-3 fatty acids, epidemiologic evidence, modest efficacy data, and low risks make omega-3 fatty acids a reasonable augmentation strategy" for the treatment of major depressive disorders (Freeman, 2010). The Task Force also found that EPA or EPD plus DHA was superior to DHA alone. Lower doses of EPA and DHA (1 gram each per day) were better than higher dose forms. Although changes in coagulation profiles would be expected in theory, they are rarely observed in practice even among patients taking anticoagulants.

St. John's Wort

In contrast, treatment of depression with St. John's wort is not recommended due to lack of efficacy in studies conducted in the United States as well as lack of quality control across various products. Substantial risk of drug–drug interactions with St. John's wort is an added concern, more so when comorbid conditions complicate the older adult's care (Freeman et al., 2010).

SAM-e

S-adenosyl methionine (SAM-e) is a naturally occurring compound that plays a role in the synthesis of neurotransmitters. Despite its theoretical appeal there is not sufficient evidence to recommend it for either sole or augmented treatment of depressive disorders in late life (Freeman et al., 2010).

Antioxidants

The theory that age-related illnesses result from oxidative stress has provoked major interest in the use of antioxidant vitamins. However, there is no clinical evidence to warrant supplementation with the antioxidant vitamins E, A, or beta-carotene (Buhr & Bales, 2010). The 2008 Cochrane review (Bjelakovic et al., 2009) found no evidence to support use of antioxidant supplements for primary or secondary disease prevention. Moreover, the reviewers found that vitamin A, beta-carotene, and vitamin E in excess may increase mortality. They warn that antioxidant supplements should be considered medicinal products and should undergo sufficient evaluation before marketing.

COUNSELING AND BEHAVIORAL INTERVENTIONS FOR A BETTER DIET

Changing a behavior pattern as personal and socially driven as diet is a major undertaking. However, the effort is likely to be successful, based on empirical evidence of persons at risk for diet-related illness. For the majority of Americans, weight increases until age 60 or 70. Once the increase has leveled off, modest changes in behavior, diet, and exercise may be quite effective. Long-term, modest gains rather than immediate, dramatic benefits are the goals. Modifications in nutritional habits are best achieved by a global, incremental approach that incorporates changes in food selection and preparation, exercise, and social reinforcers. This will make it possible to formulate a treatment plan for realistic, sustainable changes in nutritional habits. All practitioners should have the ability to educate patients and their families regarding desirable body weight and healthy proportions from the food groups, augmented by physical activity such as brisk walking.

The United States Preventive Services Task Force (2003) recommends intensive behavioral counseling for adult patients with hyperlipidemia and other known risk factors for cardiovascular and diet-related chronic disease. Although depressive disorders are not noted in the recommendation, diseases that predispose the older adult to depression are. Effective interventions include individual or group counseling delivered by nutritionists, dietitians, or specially trained primary care practitioners or health educators in the primary care setting or in other clinical settings by referral. Medium- to high-intensity counseling produces medium-to-large changes in daily intake of saturated fat, fiber, fruit, and vegetables among adult patients at increased risk for diet-related disease. Intensive interventions typically combine education with behavioral counseling over multiple sessions of 30 minutes or longer provided by a specially trained clinician.

Medium-intensity face-to-face dietary counseling is also effective, provided in two to three group or individual sessions and delivered by a nutritionist or a specially trained primary care physician or nurse practitioner. Effective lower-intensity interventions typically involve 5 minutes or less of primary care provider counseling supplemented by patient self-help materials, telephone counseling, or other interactive health communications. Most studies of these interventions have enrolled selected patients, many with diet-related risk factors such as hyperlipidemia or hypertension. Similar approaches may be effective with unselected patients, but adherence to dietary advice may be lower, and health benefits smaller, than in persons who have been told they are at higher risk for diet-related chronic disease. Office-level systems supports (prompts, reminders, and counseling algorithms) significantly improve the delivery of appropriate dietary counseling by primary care clinicians (U.S. Preventive Services Task Force, 2003; Whitlock et al., 2004).

The "Five-A" Nutrition Counseling Framework

Effective counseling combines nutritional education with targeted behavioral change to help patients acquire the support, skills, and motivation to alter eating habits and food preparation. Behaviorally oriented counseling might include teaching self-monitoring, training the patient to overcome barriers to selecting a healthy diet, helping patients to set personal goals, guidance in shopping and food preparation, and role play. Whitlock et al. (2002) describe these interventions as the "five-A" behavioral counseling framework.

1. *Assess* dietary practices and related factors. First the clinician needs to elicit a diet history that takes into account medical conditions, culture, preferences, work, and leisure activity. Who prepares the meals? What is ordered from the menu when the family dines out? Are highly glycemic refined "white foods" (bread, pasta, pastry, potatoes, rice) a major source of carbohydrates? Are "box or bag foods" with high fat and sodium (mixes, chips, sweets) a common indulgence? Are soft foods preferred due to dental problems? Brief dietary assessment questionnaires, validated for primary care settings (Calfas, Zabinski, & Rupp, 2000; Rockett & Colditz, 1997), can identify counseling needs, guide interventions, and monitor changes in patients' dietary patterns. However, they are vulnerable to respondent bias and need to be corroborated by an additional source of information when used to evaluate the efficacy of counseling (Coates et al., 1999; Kristal et al., 2000). As an alternative, patients may be asked to keep a diet diary. Simply recording the elements of each meal daily for 7 days will show patterns that can be altered or reinforced based on patient preferences.

2. *Advise* to change nutritional practices. The focus should be on food substitution to preserve health and independence rather than restriction to avoid disease. For example, patients may not be aware that increasing the proportion of fruits, vegetables, and nuts in meals will promote satiety at the same time that it enhances the quality of nutrition. Diet and exercise should be promoted as added steps toward prevention and recovery rather than something the patient "should have been doing" previously. The emphasis should be on small successes brought about by persistent effort.

3. *Agree* on personal goals for a changed diet in addition to hastening or sustaining the remission of depressive symptoms. Is weight gain or loss a priority, or is a more general healthy-aging nutritional pattern the main aim? Are elevations in serum lipids, glucose, or blood pressure salient therapeutic targets? Is there a desire to reduce the quantity of medications needed to control diabetes, hypertension, or heart disease by reducing body weight, salt intake, or highly glycemic (blood-glucose-elevating) foods?

TABLE 6.2. Simplified Dietary Recommendations for Older Adults

Nutrient	Daily amount	Sources and suggestions
Protein	12% of total calories	Fish and seafood (twice a week), poultry, eggs, low fat dairy products, legumes combined with cereals. Limit red meat to less than once a week.
Fat	30% or less of total calories	Fat is healthy if it is the right kind. Eggs, olive or canola oil, avocados, nuts should take the place of saturated oils and animal fats (butter, lard).
Carbohydrates	58% of total calories	Fruits, vegetables, legumes, whole-grain cereals should be the major component of every meal. Frozen vegetables are as nutritious as fresh. Keep fruits and nuts readily available for snacks. Avoid refined carbohydrates such as sweets and "box foods" and "if it's white, don't bite."
Folic acid	400 µg	Supplements, leafy vegetables, liver, yeast, fruits.
Vitamin D	800 IU	Supplements, fortified milk, seafood, eggs.
Calcium	1,200 mg	Supplements, dairy products, broccoli, kale, collards.
Sodium	Adequate if daily amounts above are attained	Fresh and dried herbs used instead of, or to reduce the quantity of, table salt. Minimize salty snacks and smoked, salt-cured, or salt-pickled foods.
Other vitamins, minerals, fiber, omega-3 fatty acids	Adequate if daily amounts above are attained	Adequate if dietary pattern above is sustained.

Note. Data from Rowe and Kahn (1998); Mayo Clinic Staff (2010); Buhr and Bales (2009, 2010); and National Research Council (2000).

4. *Assist* the person to change dietary practices or address motivational barriers. The "sources and suggestions" column from Table 6.2 can be copied to provide patients with simple written suggestions. Adding calcium, vitamin D, and folic acid supplements to the daily regimen is cheap and convenient and sets the stage for the more demanding changes. Substituting low-fat dairy products fortified with vitamin D for red meats will increase calcium as well as reduce fat intake. Adding more fruits and vegetables (frozen contains more vitamins than fresh) will improve vitamin, water, and fiber content of the diet and displace the more problematic items that are higher in fat and lower in fiber. Red meats and sweets are not forbidden but should not be part of every day's repast. A three-ounce serving of seafood should be consumed at least twice weekly. Seafood is the source of most of the omega-3 fatty acids found in the American diet. The National Academy of Sciences Institute of Medicine recommends selecting an array of seafood to minimize ingestion of methylmercury, which is concentrated in larger marine predators such as shark, tile fish, king mackerel, and swordfish. Like seafood, freshwater fish is also an excellent source of low-fat protein but with the exception of salmon will lack the omega-3 fatty acids found in the fattier seafoods such tuna, herring, and mackerel (Nesheim & Yaktine, 2007).

Poultry, like fish, makes a good substitute for red meat. Portion size should be controlled to approach 300 kcal per entrée (Rowe & Kahn, 1998). Success for the patient may hinge on changing the family's nutritional habits. If the Mediterranean diet makes sense, which elements would be easily adopted and which will require more effort? Take the easy steps first. Asking the person (the cook, the family) to switch to a new diet may be off-putting. Simply substituting a healthier item or increasing its frequency on the menu may seem less daunting. Self-management is the theme (American Medical Association, 2008). Pessimistic or negative comments about the feasibility of change may reflect perceptions distorted by the hopelessness of depression. As outlined in problem-solving therapy (PST), admonition and exhortation are less effective than exploration and extrapolation. Doubts about change should be examined in a nonconfrontational manner. Unrealistic goals may nonetheless have feasible components that can be prioritized. Given the goals, which obstacles (doubts) seem insurmountable and which less so? Who can help? Progress rather than perfection is the goal.

5. *Arrange* for review of dietary concerns in follow-up sessions to reinforce the initial effort, acknowledge success, modify goals, or refer the patient for more intensive counseling by a dietician or nutritionist.

For Those Who Need to Gain Weight

For severely underweight depressed persons, homemade or commercial nutritional supplements may be required, but they can provoke diarrhea due to lactose intolerance and may not be palatable. Alternatively changing to a more calorie-dense choice of offerings and adding scheduled snacks between meals should be suggested. Patients should experiment with the schedule of meals and snacks so that appetite is not suppressed. Calorie-dense foods are typically higher in fat. Their addition to meals in moderation can have a significant impact. Purposefully selecting snacks with higher fat or protein content will make every meal count. Full-fat cheeses and yogurt and avocado can be added to sandwiches. Milk can be substituted for water in soups, savory dishes, and beverages. Finger foods (sandwiches, cookies, cakes) can be made continuously available to facilitate slow but sure intake. Once desired body weight is restored, fat content can be reduced with the suggestions shown in Table 6.2.

Treatment of Overweight and Obesity

Calculation of body mass index (BMI) among persons with depression or another comorbid condition will identify those who should reduce weight for health reasons. BMI is calculated by multiplying body weight in pounds by 703 and dividing the result by height in inches squared. At 5 feet, 7 inches and 159 pounds, a person's BMI is 25. At the same height but with a weight of 191 the BMI is 30. A person with a BMI between 25 and 29 is considered at low, but not least, risk for medical comorbidities. However, those with diabetes (fasting blood sugar > 126 mg/dl), hypertension (systolic > 140, diastolic > 90), or hypercholesterolemia (high-density lipoprotein cholesterol < 35 mg/dl for men, < 45 for women) should consider treatment for overweight. Patients with a BMI greater than 29 are considered obese and in need of treatment whether or not a comorbid condition is present (National Heart, Lung and Blood Institute, 1998). Obesity is best conceptualized as a chronic illness that like diabetes or hypertension may be controlled but rarely cured. Thus the realistic goal of treatment is sustained weight reduction by 5–15% rather than a return to the lean body mass of early adult years. The goal is better function and risk reduction rather than better appearance (Bray, 1999).

Treatment of Constipation

Constipation is a frequent complaint among seniors, particularly those who have unrealistic expectations, consume little dietary fiber, take inadequate amounts of liquid, require narcotic analgesics, or do not exercise. Obviously physical activity and more fluid and fiber are the first-choice intervention. Simply increasing the amounts of fruits and vegetables will increase both fluid and fiber content. Adding one to three tablespoons of dietary fiber from psyllium will more than meet the recommendations. Bloating and cramping are less likely if the psyllium is introduced gradually. Many inexpensive preparations are available in a variety of flavors and consistencies. Patients also need to be aware that daily elimination is not the goal of good bowel hygiene.

THE EVIDENCE ON EXERCISE

The evidence supporting the physical and mental health benefits of exercise across the lifespan is compelling. Similarly, studies of successful efforts to promote increased physical activity have evolved across the range of older adult venues both community and institutionally based. Staying Healthy through Education and Prevention (STEP) offers a detailed coaching document designed to implement exercise programs in continuing care retirement communities (U.S. Department of Health and Human Services, 2011). The handouts, progressive approach, and group training sessions are ideal for professionally led community-based initiatives.

However, changes in activity habits are not easily achieved by the older individual or clinic-based practitioner. Aging "successfully" is to a large extent the result of how hard one works at it (Rowe & Kahn, 1998). Lack of physical exercise is associated with excess mortality from all causes, particularly heart disease. Although the burden of the most common chronic illnesses in America could be reduced by changes in diet and exercise (U.S. Department of Health and Human Services, 1996), these reductions depend on altered social behaviors and are not easily achieved. However, modest improvements in physical activity can have meaningful benefits for health and well-being. Even in old age, endurance, strength, and balance can be improved through exercise. The ability to educate patients and their families regarding a simple exercise program such as brisk walking is reasonable for all practitioners. More important, exercise may be seen as a universal indicator for the prevention of mental illnesses in late life, particularly the mental disorders associated with vascular diseases. To illustrate the point, Table 6.3 compares recommendations proven to prevent heart disease with those thought to lessen the risk of Alzheimer's disease. The overlap is substantial.

How Much or How Little Exercise Is Physically Beneficial?

The National Institute on Aging (1999) recommends 30 minutes of vigorous exercise daily, 7 days a week. More recent (2014) recommendations at *www.nia.nih.gov/Go4Life* offer extensive suggestions about the why and

TABLE 6.3. Recommendations for the Prevention of Heart Disease Compared to Preliminary Recommendations to Prevent Alzheimer's Disease

Heart disease[a]	Alzheimer's disease[b]
Stop smoking.	Stop smoking, avoid excess alcohol.
Exercise for 30 minutes most days if not every day.	Exercise both the mind and body; stay socially engaged.
If hypertensive, get treated; if diabetic, lower your blood sugar through diet, exercise, medications if needed.	Minimize any risks of heart disease and stroke.
Use diet and exercise to achieve and maintain a healthy body weight.	Keep body weight within healthy guidelines.
Use diet, exercise, and medications if needed to lower your cholesterol.	If elevated, lower your cholesterol.
Limit consumption of animal fats, *trans* fats, starches, and sugar.	Take steps to avoid falls and head injury.
Eat lots of whole grains and whole-grain products, high-fiber fruits and vegetables ("if it's white, don't bite").	Increase your intake of dark-skinned fruits and vegetables, cold-water fish, and nuts (walnuts, pecans, almonds).

[a]Data from Torpy, Burke, and Glass (2009).
[b]Data from *www.alz.org/alzheimers_disease_causes_risk_factors.asp#other* (retrieved March 23, 2014).

how of exercise in old age. Manson et al. (1999) found that 3 hours of brisk walking weekly conferred similar benefits compared to more vigorous exercise. The investigators found that women who began exercising only in midlife also achieved substantial benefit. Over 8 years of observation, the benefits amounted to a 30 to 40% reduction in coronary events among more than 70,000 women ages 40 to 65 years. The benefits remained substantial even after correcting for age, illness, and lifestyle differences in the participants. The intensity and amount of exercise also has an impact on insulin sensitivity and atherosclerosis (Mayer-Davis et al., 1998). Because most older adults get less than the recommended level of exercise, the percentage of coronary events that are potentially preventable if the exercise guidelines were universally applied is nearly 50% (Stofan et al., 1998). The size of associated reductions in the prevalence of vascular depression and vascular dementia is uncertain but not to be ignored.

Exercise and Mood Disorders

The Cochrane Systematic Review (Cooney et al., 2014) found exercise moderately more effective than control interventions for reducing symptoms of depression but no more effective than pharmacological or psychological therapies. The review noted the difficulty of blinding both those receiving and those delivering and assessing the intervention. Also noted were the surprisingly small number of trials. Missing were any comparisons of exercise as an augmenting intervention for psychotherapy or pharmacotherapy. Studies examined below illustrate both the promise and problems of seeking to measure the benefits of exercise for depression.

Singh, Clements, and Fiatarone (1997) conducted a 10-week study of 32 persons ages 60–84 with major or minor depression or dysthymia randomized to progressive resistance training or attention control. Measures of depression, pain, and social functioning were all significantly improved among the exercise group compared to control participants with intensity of training being the major predictor of the reduction in depression. Subsequently Singh-Manoux et al. (2005) randomized 60 community-residing adults with major or minor depression to high-intensity or low-intensity weight training or routine care by general practitioners. The weight training was supervised and performed three times weekly for 8 weeks. Reductions in HAM-D scores of 50% were achieved among 61% of the high-intensity, 29% of the low-intensity, and 21% of the routine care groups.

Using a cross-sectional community survey of more than 40,000 adults ages 18–89 (more than 20% of the sample were 60 years of age or older), Harvey et al. (2010) found an inverse relationship between the amount of leisure-time physical activity and diagnosis-level symptoms of depression. This cross-sectional association was present with leisure-time but not workplace activity and did not depend on the intensity of activity. Whether the activity was light or intense, persons practicing 3 or more hours per week halved their odds of being depressed. Those with 1–2 hours per week did nearly as well. And the size and significance of the effects remained when results were adjusted for age. Higher levels of social support and social engagement were more important in explaining the relationship between leisure activity and depression than biological changes such resting pulse (parasympathetic vagal tone) and metabolic markers (glucose, cholesterol, triglycerides, BMI). The effects were significant for both low- and high-intensity activities, the latter defined as those which caused sweating or shortness of breath.

There is also a modest but generally positive literature on exercise for anxiety disorders (Strohle et al., 2005; Dunn, Trivedi, & Neal, 2001) and sleep disturbances (King et al., 1997, 2000). Physical activity at various levels of intensity results in improvements in perceived stress, anxiety, and well-being (U.S. Department of Health and Human Services, 1996). Benefits are achieved through a reduction in physical disability and through improved self-image, sense of mastery, and simple enjoyment. Exercise, both aerobic and anaerobic, is an effective adjunct treatment for anxiety. Exercise alone is less effective than antidepressant medication but adds to the impact of group CBT for social phobias (Jayakody, Gunadasa, & Hosker, 2014).

Exercise and Cognitive Function

A positive relationship between physical activity and cognitive function is evident in most (Achana et al., 2005; Abbott et al., 2004; Fritsch et al., 2005; Malmstrom et al., 2005; Ghisletta, Bickel, & Lövden, 2006; Chan et al., 2005) but not all (Verghese et al., 2003) observational studies and in a number of experimental investigations (Colcombe et al., 2006; Colcombe & Kramer, 2003; Kramer et al., 1999). In a study by Colcombe et al. (2006), 59 sedentary but healthy community volunteers ages 60–79 were randomized to either an aerobic exercise group or a stretching and muscle toning group. Participants in both the toning/stretching and aerobic exercise groups attended three exercise sessions weekly for 6 months with attendance exceeding 85% for both groups. As flexibility increased in the toning/stretching group, stretches of increasing difficulty were introduced. Exercise intensity targets for the aerobic group were based on peak heart rate observed during graded exercise testing, with the initial training target being 40–50% of peak rate and the final target being 60–70%. Both groups completed graded exercise testing at baseline and 6 months afterward to determine peak oxygen uptake (VO_{2peak}). In addition, magnetic resonance images of both gray and white matter were obtained for both groups before and after 6 months of intervention as well as for 20 younger persons (ages 18–30) who were also observed but without intervention.

At the outset there were no significant differences between the groups on demographic, health, or cognitive measures, or on VO_{2peak}. However, after 6 months the aerobic group had increased their VO_{2peak} by 16.1% compared to a 5.3% increase in the toning/stretching group. More important, the aerobic group had significantly increased brain volume in the prefrontal and temporal cortices and anterior white matter subtending the anterior third of the corpus callosum. Of note, these regions are associated with age-related decline in attentional control and memory. The findings are all the more noteworthy in that study participants who were healthy and well educated experienced an exercise-related increase in brain volume as opposed to the expected age-related decrease.

Erickson et al. (2011) found that exercise training increased the size of the hippocampus and improved memory in association with increased plasma levels of BDNF. At baseline, 6 months, and 12 months, magnetic resonance imaging, BDNF, and a spatial memory task were assessed to measure the effects of three 40-minute supervised physical activity sessions per week for 1 year. The participants were sedentary older adults with mean ages of 67 for the experimental and 65 for the comparison group. More than 60% of the participants were women. Sixty individuals were randomized to aerobic exercise consisting of walking with progressive intensity to reach a targeted percentage of baseline $VO_{2\,max}$. The comparison group did a variety of static stretching and toning activities of progressively increasing intensity. Compared to the stretching and toning group, the exercise group increased their VO_2 by 7.78% versus 1.11%.

These studies are also consistent with animal research findings of increased hippocampal neurogenesis (Trejo, Carro, & Torres-Aleman, 1996) and enhanced learning (Swinburn et al., 1998; Anderson et al.,

2000) associated with exercise. And they are intriguing given the relationship between loss of hippocampal volume and depression (Vasic et al., 2008). These data suggest that in addition to comparing the brain to a computer that can be upgraded with education, it should also be thought of as a muscle that can be strengthened with physical exercise. When mental and physical exercises are combined, the result is measurable benefit in both cognition and physical function (Law et al., 2014).

MOTIVATING PATIENTS TO EXERCISE

Resnick and Spellbring (2000) advocate a seven-step approach to motivate older persons to exercise. First educate both patient and family caregivers about the benefits of exercise and what to expect. The emphasis is placed on regular physical activity rather than calisthenics or sports play, which seniors often associate with the word exercise. Pointing out the immediate benefits for activities of daily living and for interaction with grandchildren will be more motivating than promises of disease reduction or a longer life. Heavy breathing and sweating are normal responses and indicate that the activity is having a beneficial effect. However, dizziness or chest tightness or pain are warning signs and call for a pause if not a complete halt. Exercise has an alerting effect that may interfere with sleep if performed in the evening.

Second, prescreening is generally unnecessary for low-intensity activity (60% of maximum heart rate) or moderate-intensity (80% of maximum heart rate) exercise. Examples of moderate-intensity activities include raking leaves for 30 minutes or walking 1.75 miles in 35 minutes. Exercise stress testing is rarely indicated, but checking the patient's pulse and blood pressure will have a reassuring effect.

Third, identify and use short- and long-term goals to initiate as well as to reward activity. Goals must be achievable but challenging enough to extend beyond the present level of daily activity. Short-term goals focus on achieving the target exercise duration or intensity such as walking 15 minutes before stopping to rest. Longer-term goals focus on the ultimate benefits, such as being able to visit friends or family whose homes have stairs.

Fourth, exposure to some form of exercise activity will build confidence and reinforce regular activity. Is there a partner available to reinforce the effort? Simple maneuvers such as recommending that the older couple exercise together may provide important reinforcement.

A morning routine of exercise is more easily sustained than one in the afternoon or evening. However, exercise in the morning routine may require a longer warm-up period. Approach barriers to exercise with problem solving. Common barriers and solutions as developed by Resnick (2003) are listed in Table 6.4.

Fifth, the identification of role models who can champion the benefits of exercise either in the community or the facility adds the element of peer support. Suggest the patient join an exercise class or approach a resident of the facility who is a regular exerciser. Exercise partners reinforce motivation.

Sixth, practitioners can reinforce patients by reassuring them that they are capable of both initiating and sustaining regular physical activity. Prescribe a brief telephone contact after exercise; this will indicate a positive expectation and genuine interest on the part of the practitioner. Seventh, identify rewards for goals attained. Reinforcing the older adult's sense of self-efficacy and providing emotional support may prove to be substantial contributors to physical activity and functional independence (Seeman et al., 1995). Verbal praise and expressions of admiration from the practitioner can be powerful motivators. In long-term care settings, a surprise visit to the exercise session will demonstrate the importance of the activity to the prescriber and thereby the facility resident.

HOW TO PRESCRIBE EXERCISE

Exercise may be preventative in some instances, but the primary care clinician is most often caring for older adults with illness already present. Thus an exercise prescription must be tailored to fit social circumstances and physical capacity. Again, long-term incremental gains are the goal rather than sudden, dramatic change. This will make it possible to formulate a treatment plan for realistic, sustainable changes in activity patterns. Although adults may voice excuses for not exercising, it is the practitioner's lack of knowledge about how to prescribe exercise that is the greater obstacle (Swinburn et al., 1998). The clinician first needs to elicit an exercise history that takes into account medical conditions, culture, preferences, work, recreational opportunities, and leisure activities. A prescription that emphasizes the social rewards and physical pleasures of exercise will lead to more lasting changes than a regimen focused on discipline and hard work. Was the person athletic

TABLE 6.4. Problem Solving for Barriers to (and Excuses Not to) Exercise

Barrier/excuse	Solution
"I'm too old."	You're never too old to improve your physical health and mental well-being with exercise.
"Why bother? How much time do I have left anyway?"	Exercise may not add years to your life, but it will add life to your years through improved health and independence.
"I'm too fat."	Being overweight is one of the best reasons to increase physical activity. Low-intensity exercise such as walking is safe even if you are overweight.
"I'll get injured."	Lack of physical activity injures your muscles, bones, and joints. Low-impact activities such as walking or swimming are safe.
"I'll fall."	Because exercise builds both strength and balance, it is one of the best ways to reduce your risk of falling. Hold on to the kitchen sink to exercise the lower extremities or use assistive devices such as a chair, cane, or walker for added security.
"It will hurt."	Exercise lessens the pain of osteoarthritis and osteoporosis. Use assistive devices to protect vulnerable areas. Use an analgesic before the exercise session.
"I'll get too tired."	Exercise actually increases perceived levels of energy. You can rest before or after exercise to counter worries of excessive fatigue.
"There's no safe place in my neighborhood; it's too hot or too cold."	Walk the halls or stair wells in your apartment building. Exercise with a partner. Find a climate-controlled shopping mall for walking.
"It is too boring."	Find a physical activity you enjoy and do it with a friend. Listen to music, radio, or books on tape while you exercise.
"I haven't the time."	Make your health and the enjoyment of exercise a priority. Reassess your schedule and allot 30 minutes per day. It is easier to sustain if it is scheduled first thing in the morning.

Note. Adapted from Kennedy (2007b). Adapted with permission from *Primary Psychiatry.*

in youth? Were group sports the only exercise outlet? Are safe, easily accessed parks, walkways, or climate-controlled shopping malls conducive to walking available?

The biomechanical and motivational components of the exercise prescription are summarized in Table 6.5. The traditional three components of exercise are flexibility, strength, and endurance. But for older adults in particular, balance, injury prevention, persistence, and reinforcement are critical to an optimal exercise prescription. A progressive exercise prescription is provided in Figure 6.1, but it must be tailored from the outset to the patient's interests, motivation, and fitness potential. Walking 30 minutes on most days of the week should be sufficient to achieve substantial health benefits (Stofan et al., 1998). For seniors who are especially cautious, a 20-minute walk three times a week may be sufficient to begin. To reduce risk and fear of falls, add the first three steps of tai chi, "sun rising," "step right," and "step left," which incorporate the postural awareness, balance, and quadriceps strengthening of the long form but are easier to learn (Yan, 1999; Sattin et al., 2005). Sink-side balance exercises illustrated in the STEP implementation guide (U.S. Department of Health and Human Services, 2011) may be used to build confidence as well.

Instructions for pain-free stretching and range of motion exercises can be found in most exercise books and fitness magazines. It is important to emphasize that stretching should come after the exercise rather than before. Stretching must also be introduced gradually to joints and muscles that have lost their elasticity with age and inactivity. For optimal benefit a daily routine incorporating 30–45 minutes of endurance exercise with twice-weekly resistance (weight) training will be needed (Welle, 1998). Both the lifting and lowering of the weight should be done in "slow motion" for maximum effect. Hypertension is not a contraindication to strength training. Indeed, diastolic pressures will decrease (2–3 mm Hg) over a 4-week period of 3 sessions per week (Brandon, Sharon, & Boyette, 1997). Neither is diabetes a contraindication: exercise lowers blood sugar by increasing insulin sensitivity (Mayer-Davis et al., 1998).

Highly motivated individuals and those with an athletic background may seek to play sports but will need time and effort to regain reasonable fitness and avoid injury. Supervised exercise though a health club or exercise group may be preferred for the solitary senior or one whose spouse or family does not "believe in" exercise. Although only half of those who start structured exercise are likely to continue for 15 months, increases in strength and coordination will remain above

TABLE 6.5. Biomechanical and Motivation Components of the Exercise Prescription for Older Persons

Component	Methods	Goal	Benefits	Target condition
Flexibility	Daily graduated stretching without pain, warm up first	Increased range of motion	Lessened disability, pain reduction, contracture prevention, improved gait, improved sexual performance	Arthritis, pain, immobility, falls and gait disturbance, stroke rehabilitation
Strength	Weight-bearing exercise, tai chi, mechanized resistance training	Increased muscle strength and mass	Fewer falls, better cardiovascular performance, better ambulation, reduced medications for diabetes, improved mood	Depression, diabetes, MI or stroke rehabilitation, Parkinson's disease, gait disturbance, falls, osteoporosis
Endurance	Walking, swimming, cycling, running, tennis, basketball	Greater stamina at all levels of functioning	Weight loss, better cognitive, cardiovascular, and sexual performance, improved mood and sleep, reduced medications for diabetes, angina, hypertension	Depression, anxiety, panic, sleep disturbance, cognitive impairment, diabetes, angina, obesity, hypertension, MI or stroke rehabilitation, chronic lung disease

Injury prevention	Warm-up, moderation, consistency, progressive increase in duration and effort, proper footwear, clothing, and equipment	Preservation of consistent exercise routine, prevention of pain and disability, resiliency	All of the above	Arthritis, podiatric conditions
Balance	Postural awareness, tai chi, dance or movement therapy	Safer exercise and activities of daily living	Reduced risk of falls	Stroke, Parkinson's disease, gait disturbance
Persistence	Daily routine, variety, cross-training, group training	Stretching and endurance work daily, strengthening and balance every other day, fatigue not pain	All of the above	All of the above
Reinforcement	Recreational rather than therapeutic attitude, group training, convenience, low cost, written prescription, follow-up	Pleasure, socialization, motivation, pride in one's appearance, maintenance of gains and goals	All of the above	All of the above

Note. Adapted from Kennedy (2000). Copyright 2000 by The Guilford Press. Adapted by permission.

The general rules are: (1) Start slowly—give yourself 12 weeks to get in condition; (2) if one exercise hurts, substitute one that does not; (3) track your progress; (4) light exercise you like is better than a heavy routine you loathe; (5) do not give up—persistence leads to success.

How to use this chart: (1) Record your baseline level of physical activity over an average week. For example, write the number of stair flights you climbed or minutes you spent walking or the approximate weight of packages you carried. (2) Underline the physical activities you feel safe performing. (3) Begin exercising every other day at a relaxed pace. At the end of the first week, record the minutes or amount of exercise you completed. (4) In the second week, exert slightly more effort but do not increase the amount. (5) In the third week, begin exercising for 5 days but do not increase the effort. (6) Starting with week 4, increase the days per week of exercise to 7; add effort only if you feel like it. (7) By the end of week 12, you should be exercising half an hour for 5–7 days per week. Now review your progress and set goals for staying fit or exercising even more. A little exercise goes a long way, but more exercise is better.

Purpose	Type of physical activity	Duration, intensity, baseline	Duration, intensity, week 1	Duration, intensity, week 2	Duration, intensity, week 3	Duration, intensity, week 12
To establish your routine level of physical activity	Walking, housekeeping, gardening, sports					
To warm up, prevent injury, improve balance and posture	Slow walking or range of motion exercises, postural awareness, tai chi (first three steps)					
To increase endurance	Brisk walking, sports					
To increase strength	Stair climbing, chair squats, biceps curls, triceps extensions, sit-ups, resistance training, tai chi (long form)					
To relax, cool down, increase flexibility	Slow walking followed by gentle stretching, range of motion exercises					

FIGURE 6.1. Progressive exercise prescription. Adapted from Kennedy (2000). Copyright 2000 by The Guilford Press. Adapted by permission.

baseline measures (Boyette, Sharon, & Brandon, 1997). Among nursing home residents, weight training three times per week for 8 weeks doubled strength and increased walking speed by 50%. These gains were sustained with only one weekly weight-training session (Fiatarone et al., 1994). Programs incorporating strength, flexibility, balance, and endurance can be administered to groups including frail, cognitively impaired, or incontinent residents and are more likely to preserve physical function than simple range of motion exercise (Darien-Alexis et al., 1999). Some form of exercise from range of motion to competitive sports should be available to almost every senior.

CONCLUSION

Modest improvements in diet and physical activity can have major effects on the health and well-being of older adults, both in preventing disease and modifying the severity of illness after onset. Improvements in diet and physical activity to lessen depression make good common sense and have theoretical appeal and empirical support. Brief counseling for the patient and whoever prepares the meals to promote a Mediterranean dietary pattern supplemented with vitamin D is a straightforward means of reducing age- and illness-related risk factors for depression. The clinician's attention to both the biomechanics and motivational components of exercise can increase adherence to healthy behavior by ensuring that increased physical activity is rewarding in and of itself. This requires realistic expectations, a long-term orientation, and urging that exercise be a social rather than solitary pursuit. That physical activity and a better diet mean better health will hardly be a surprise to the older person. But it may be surprising for practitioners that they should be considered routine elements in the behavioral activation approach to combating depression. Knowledgeable and optimistic practitioners may be the critical motivators for improved diet and physical activity for depressed persons at any age.

CHAPTER 7

Electroconvulsive Therapy

Convulsive therapies have a centuries-long history in the practice of medicine, starting with seizures induced by camphor, then insulin and now electricity (Fink, 1984). Overshadowed by advances in pharmacotherapy and sensationalized in the popular media, ECT remains an important therapeutic modality even if it is most often considered a treatment of last resort. What follows is meant to provide the practitioner with a realistic appraisal of indications, risks, and benefits of ECT for the older patient. The intent is not instruction in the practice of ECT but rather the means to prepare patients and their family members to consider ECT when depressive illness has become life threatening, grossly disabling, or refractory to other therapies. Kitty Dukakis's memoir (Dukakis & Tye, 2006) of her experience with ECT is forthright and may be recommended to patients and family members who want an accessible source of information. A celebrity openly discussing an illness can make the patient feel less embarrassed and more willing to consider the treatment (Whooley, 2012).

WHAT IS ECT AND HOW IS THE TREATMENT PERFORMED?

ECT is the most highly effective therapy currently available for severe major depression (Unützer & Park, 2012). The treatment consists of electricity applied to the scalp crossing the brain, inducing a seizure. Because ECT is performed under general anesthesia patients are evaluated by an anesthesiologist for pulmonary and cardiovascular risk as well as potential complications from medication (Tess & Smetana, 2009). Consultation from a cardiologist will also be required when coronary artery disease, heart valve pathology, a pacemaker, or an implanted cardioverter are present. These consultants do not "clear" the patient for the procedure but rather advise on measures to reduce risk and on the need for any additional diagnostic studies. Brain imaging with computed tomography or magnetic resonance imaging is not considered routine (Lisanby, 2007). Medications such as lithium, theophylline, benzodiazepines, and anticonvulsants are tapered or withdrawn prior to treatment, but antidepressants may be continued. In the 12 hours before treatment the patient takes nothing by mouth with the exception of critical medications such as antihypertensives and insulin. Immediately prior to treatment, leads for the electrocardiogram and electroencephalogram are attached to the patient in addition to a blood pressure cuff and finger pulse oximeter. This allows the anesthesiologist to continuously monitor heart rate, blood pressure, oxygen saturation, and respiration and enables the psychiatrist to confirm the occurrence of a convulsion.

An intravenous line is placed and the short-acting barbiturate thiopental sodium is used to induce anesthesia. Mask ventilation with supplemental oxygen is used rather than intubation once the patient is unconscious. A beta-blocking agent (labetalol or esmolol) may be administered to reduce the hypertension, tachycardia, and cardiac conduction abnormalities that result from the sympathetic discharge that occurs during the seizure. However, Tess and Smetana (2009) warn against routine use of beta-blockers, citing shortened seizure duration and reduced ECT efficacy as possible complications. Glycopyrrolate or atropine may be used to minimize reflex bradycardia and excess salivation. Once anesthetized the patient is given the rapid-acting neuromuscular blocking agent succinylcholine to prevent muscle contractions that would otherwise result from the seizure.

Two electrodes are then placed in the right unilateral (over the vertex and temporal area) or bilateral (bitemporal) positions to deliver the electrical stimulus. Right unilateral placement is associated with less postseizure confusion and amnesia but is less effective than bilateral placement (Sackeim et al., 1993). During the initial session a subthreshold stimulus may be escalated until a seizure results. This provides the mark for subsequent treatments, in which a percentage of the threshold stimulus will be administered to reliably induce the convulsion. An age-adjusted algorithm may also be used to approximate the threshold initially, but in as much as age is a minor determinant of seizure threshold, dose escalation may be required. The dose of electricity delivered to induce the seizure is measured in millicoulombs. To be considered adequate the seizure should last a minimum of 25 seconds as observed on the EEG (Sackeim et al., 2009). Treatments will number 6–12, usually given every other weekday or less frequently depending of the severity of associated cognitive impairment. Treatments may be limited to twice weekly and applied unilaterally to the nondominant hemisphere to minimize confusion. Patients are expected to be awake and alert 30 to 60 minutes following the treatment, but mild confusion or slowed cognition may persist between treatments, not fully resolving until past the time of hospital discharge.

HOW DOES ECT WORK?

Understanding of ECT's therapeutic mechanism of action remains elusive. ECT produces changes in neurotransmitter activity and density as well as increasing the array and concentration of neurotransmitters. It increases serotonergic activity as well as cortical GABA concentrations. ECT results in substantial down regulation of beta-adrenergic receptors. Based on animal data, enhanced noradrenergic transmission following ECT ameliorates adverse cognitive effects (Sackeim et al., 2009). ECT also impacts the hypothalamic–pituitary–adrenal axis, normalizing the hypercortisolemia seen in some depressed patients. Functional brain activation is altered, and hippocampal neurogenesis is enhanced following ECT. Synaptic plasticity and neuronal structure are also modified. However, beyond the neural and neurohumoral explanations are data suggesting that late-life depression is related to dysfunction in the frontal–striatal–limbic circuitry due to vascular lesions in the prefrontal white matter. A "disconnection syndrome" results, with both cortical and limbic structures "shorting out," causing impairments in mood, thinking, and executive function and poor response to antidepressant medications (Lisanby, 2007). The circuitry metaphor lends itself to the notion that ECT "reboots" the brain to break the cycle of depression. This may be as helpful an explanation as any other but remains metaphorical at best.

WHEN IS ECT INDICATED AND IS IT EVER THE TREATMENT OF CHOICE?

Especially for older patients, practitioners will exhaust alternatives before recommending this treatment. Nonetheless, the suggestion that ECT may be necessary should be made before patient and family are exhausted as well. Compassion dictates immunizing the patient and family early on to lessen the reaction when ECT is recommended as the best if not the only choice available. Lisanby (2007) summarizes recommendations from the American Psychiatric Association Task Force on ECT as well as the United Kingdom's National Institute for Clinical Evidence (UK ECT Review Group, 2003). Both groups recommend ECT for severe depression after other treatments have failed, but only the American Psychiatric Association suggests ECT for the prevention of recurrent depression. Lisanby adds that prior beneficial response to ECT may make it a first choice as well, particularly if distress or disabilities are severe.

For patients so severely disturbed that they refuse life-saving medications (insulin, antiarrhythmics) or cannot control suicidal intent or violent outbursts, ECT may be the most effective option (Lisanby, 2007; Sackeim & Prudic, 2005). It is especially useful in cases of medication inefficacy or intolerance or when food and fluids are refused. Patients with delusional depression may demonstrate paranoia about their food, medications, or caregivers, precluding pharmacological treatment. The choice of ECT over aggressive pharmacotherapy is made by weighing the risks of prolonged suffering and uncertainty that medication will work against the burden of hospital treatment, medical conditions that may complicate general anesthesia, and fears of the patient and family. After a course of ECT, patients should be treated with continuation pharmacotherapy following recovery (Sackeim et al., 2001). Patients who have failed to benefit from intensive antidepressant treatment before receiving ECT have lower acute response rates and are more likely to relapse subsequently, even when antidepressant continuation treatment with a new medication is provided. Maintenance ECT, a single treatment given at monthly intervals, is sometimes used to prevent relapse, but the burden placed on patients and their families may limit its usefulness for the long-term management of late-life major depression (Kellner et al., 2006).

ECT is generally considered the treatment of choice for major depression with psychosis (Parker et al., 1992), but combination antipsychotic and antidepressant regimens have emerged that rival the efficacy if not the rapid onset of ECT's effects. Meyers et al. (2009) randomized 259 adults with psychotic depression to a double-blind regimen of olanzapine plus sertraline or olanzapine plus placebo. The mean age of the 142 participants ages 60 and over was 71.7 years. More than 70% of the participants were hospitalized at the time of the study. The mean dose of olanzapine for the 60 and over group was 13.5 mg (*SD* 5.1); for sertraline the mean was 165 mg (*SD* 43.7). Over the 12 weeks of the study, the remission rate for the combined olanzapine/sertraline group was 41.9% compared to 23.9% for olanzapine monotherapy. By week 2, 10% had remitted; by week 4, the number rose to 20%. Of note, rates of remission and tolerability were similar between the younger and older groups. Both groups experienced significant increases in serum cholesterol and triglycerides. Only the younger group experienced significant elevations in fasting blood glucose. Although both young and old gained significant amounts of weight, the mean gain among the younger participants was double that of the older (14 vs. 7 pounds). Thus olanzapine combined with sertraline, at substantial but tolerable doses, offers an alternative to ECT that may be preferred by some patients and their families and practitioners. Nevertheless, most patients in the study did not achieve remission despite the intensive treatment afforded by hospitalization. For those who did, the time to remission was prolonged compared to studies of ECT for psychotic depression (Petrides et al., 2001). And the adverse metabolic effects of olanzapine are troublesome. These data can help all concerned weigh the risk, burden, and benefits of ECT over aggressive pharmacotherapy.

BENEFITS OF ECT

The principal benefits of ECT are the speed with which it achieves remission and the success rate with severe depression. The efficacy of ECT approaches a response rate of 90% when bilateral ECT is administered in academic centers, but less in other settings (Prudic et al., 2004). Single-treatment maintenance ECT can be administered as an outpatient procedure in ambulatory surgery settings over intervals of several weeks to months (Hay et al., 1990) and offers rates of sustained recovery comparable to maintenance antidepressant therapy (Kellner et al., 2006). The Consortium for Research in ECT (Husain et al., 2004), in a prospective study of 253, patients found that over half experienced a

50% reduction in symptoms within the first week or the third treatment with ECT. By the 10th treatment (week 3 or 4) 65% achieved remission. With additional treatments 75% reached remission. More important, of those ages 65 and over, 90% achieved remission (O'Connor et al., 2001). Stated differently, in the first week of treatment most patients were better and by the fourth week most were well.

More recent data suggest that antidepressant medications administered concurrently with ECT improve remission rates. In a larger-scale study of patients with major depressive disorder, all participants received either high-dose right unilateral or routine bilateral ECT. Psychotropic medications were withdrawn prior to the initiation of treatment. To determine the risks and benefits of concurrent antidepressant pharmacotherapy, venlafaxine, nortriptyline, or placebo were added after the first ECT. Doses were escalated to a target of 100–120 ng/ml blood level of nortriptyline or a total 225 mg per day of venlafaxine. Persons judged to be frail received a lower starting dose and more gradual escalation. Patients receiving nortriptyline experienced a 15% increase in remission rate above that observed with placebo. Administration of venlafaxine also achieved a superior remission rate but less substantial than that seen with nortriptyline. Right unilateral treatment at six times the seizure threshold was as effective as bilateral treatment at 1.5 times threshold. Post-ECT declines in global cognitive performance, memory, and learning, working memory, and recall of autobiographical events were observed across all combinations of treatment. Advancing age was associated with greater deficits. However, global performance, memory, and learning and working memory were significantly less impaired among patients receiving nortriptyline. Retrograde and anterograde amnesia were both less substantial among those who received right unilateral therapy (Sackeim et al., 2009).

RISKS AND BURDENS OF ECT

Age-related factors increase the value of ECT for geriatric mental disorders but also increase the likelihood of adverse reactions. This paradox is explained by the higher response rates among older adults, along with the greater prevalence of age-related illnesses such as diabetes, hypertension, and heart disease. Not surprisingly, cardiovascular complications are the most frequent adverse events associated with ECT (Huang et al., 1989). Dolenc et al. (2004) described the experience of 29 patients,

26 with pacemakers and 3 with implantable cardioverter defibrillators, all of whom received ECT and benefited from the treatment. Only one serious cardiac event occurred, an episode of supraventricular tachycardia that resolved in the intensive cardiac care unit. Following resolution of the tachycardia, the patient completed the course of ECT without incident. Having reviewed data from 1984 to 1994, Kramer (1999) concluded that the death rate associated with ECT was 0.19 per 10,000 treatments.

Although there are reports of manic reactions to ECT among older persons (Serby, 2001), the cognitive side effects of ECT are the principal factor limiting its acceptance. The cognitive impairment associated with ECT includes temporary postseizure confusion, transient anterograde and retrograde amnesia, and less commonly a permanent amnestic syndrome in which events surrounding the treatment are forgotten (Gardner & O'Connor, 2008). Initially anterograde amnesia or the inability to learn new information may be pronounced, particularly during bilateral ECT, but it improves rapidly following completion of treatment. A program of cognitive remediation similar to that used for persons with seizure disorders has been developed to preserve memories, which are usually compromised following ECT (Choi et al., 2011). The full extent of cognitive recovery may not be evident until weeks to months following treatment (Sackeim et al., 2007). Although patients may complain that ECT has had a long-term effect on memory, longitudinal studies have failed to demonstrate lasting cognitive effects; furthermore, improved memory, perhaps owing to recovery from depression, has been reported. Indeed, memory complaints may reflect the residue of depression more than the aftereffects of ECT (Prudic, Peyser, & Sackeim, 2000). Thus the presence of dementia should not be considered a contraindication to ECT.

There are few absolute medical contraindications other than the presence of increased intracranial pressure or unstable angina. Patients with coronary artery disease or cerebral vascular disease may safely be administered ECT through the use of pharmacological management for the autonomic responses that may occur during treatment. Nevertheless, a recent myocardial infarction or cerebral vascular event and unstable coronary artery disease increase the risk of complications. In summary, the principal risks of ECT are cardiovascular, and the principal burdens of ECT are those associated with hospitalization and transient impairments in cognition.

INFORMED CONSENT FOR ECT

Compared to many medical or surgical procedures, obtaining informed consent for ECT differs in several significant ways. Although less so than consent for vital organ transplantation, the ECT consent process and associated documentation are complex and extensive. For example, consent is sought for a course of treatment, not a single episode. Depression and psychosis have an impact on the patient's initial decision, and the posttreatment delirium will complicate subsequent consent as well. Nonetheless, psychosis, depression, or even involuntary hospitalization do not of themselves preclude sufficient understanding to consent. Although the individual must give consent, family involvement is the expected norm. The physician provides details about risks, both cognitive and medical, electrode placement, stimulus dosing, anesthesia and related restrictions, preparation for the procedure, and the course of treatment. As treatment proceeds, the physician and patient discuss the benefits and burdens of treatment and any changes in the procedure that may be indicated. As a result, consent is an ongoing, interactive process. Consent is deemed adequate when sufficient information about the treatment has been conveyed and when the patient or surrogate consenter is documented to be capable of understanding and acting upon the information. The physician offering the treatment seeks to persuade the patient, but not to the extent that a reasonable observer or family member would view the process as coercive. Ambivalence and indecisiveness may be part of the illness and need to be addressed therapeutically. Respect for autonomy does not include abandoning the patient to an impaired or ill-informed decision. Patients vary widely in their capacity to incorporate details of treatment, so the presentation should be tailored to the person's educational background, vocabulary, and intelligence. Comprehension is aided when family are present, when the material is presented across several iterations, and when written material is used as an adjunct, not a substitute, for an open discussion (Kellner et al., 2012). Obviously, practitioners who do not administer the treatment are not equipped to provide information on which consent is based. Nonetheless, they can convey support and compassion by discussing the "big picture" of indications, reducing the fears and stigma associated with the treatment, and assuring patient and family that the recommendation is a request for a consultation rather than an abandonment. Proper preparation is key to enhancing the patient's capacity to decide.

Finally, patients and their family members may have questions about transcranial magnetic stimulation as an alternative to ECT. Transcranial magnetic stimulation is delivered by positioning a magnetic coil over the scalp above the left prefrontal cortex. It does not require anesthesia and does not provoke a seizure or amnesia but requires 20 to 30 administrations spaced over 4 to 6 weeks. There are a number of studies comparing transcranial magnetic stimulation to ECT. ECT achieves higher remission rates and older adults are less likely to benefit from transcranial stimulation (Taylor, 2014).

CONCLUSION

The possibility that ECT will be required should be presented early rather than late in treatment of depression complicated by psychosis, suicidal intent, or refusal of life-saving medication or nutrition. The patient and family should be informed that the acute confusion induced by ECT is certain to occur but resolves with time. The risk of a stroke or heart attack due to the cardiovascular effects of the seizure or the anesthesia is elevated among persons with cardiovascular or cerebrovascular disease but can be minimized with pretreatment medications and careful monitoring during treatment by the attending anesthesiologist. These potential risks should be weighed against (1) the near certainty that without ECT, full recovery from antidepressant-refractory depression complicated by psychosis or suicidal ideation is unlikely in the extreme, and (2) the high probability that the person will respond within the first week and achieve remission within the third week of treatment with ECT. Indications for ECT, as well as its risks, burdens, and benefits, are summarized in Table 7.1.

TABLE 7.1. Summary of Indications for ECT as Well as Risks, Burdens, and Benefits

Indications	Risks	Burdens	Benefits
1. Major depressive disorder, severe, complicated by psychosis, risk of suicide, violence, or other life-threatening behavior (refusal of medications, food, or fluids) 2. Bipolar depression 3. Prevention of recurrent depression 4. Treatment of recurrent depressive episode when past episodes have responded to ECT 5. Depression refractory to antidepressant therapy	1. Cardiac arrhythmia, infarction (elevated by recent myocardial infarction, unstable angina) 2. Stroke (elevated with increased intracranial pressure or recent stroke) 3. Comorbid physical illness rather than age elevates risk	1. Hospitalization 2. Anesthesia 3. Postictal confusion 4. Anterograde and/or retrograde amnesia 5. Stigma, fear	1. Highest probability of remission of any available treatment for mood disorders 2. Induces more rapid and reliable response than psychotherapy or pharmacotherapy

CHAPTER 8

Reducing the Risk of Suicide in Late Life

Crude death rates due to suicide have declined over the last five decades, but the number of deaths is expected to rise with the increasing number of older Americans. Although there is no evidence to support universal screening for suicidal ideation (Haney et al., 2012), consensus is emerging on the need to develop a broadly based public health approach to preventing suicidal behavior, driven in part by startlingly high suicide rates among U.S. active-duty personnel and veterans of the wars in Afghanistan and Iraq. This chapter first reviews suicide rates and risk factors for older adults and then discusses population-based approaches for reducing the risk of suicidal behavior in older persons.

SUICIDE RATES AMONG OLDER ADULTS

Table 8.1 shows suicide rates among adults ages 65 and older from 1960 to 2010. Across the six decades, the highest rate was 24.5 per 100,000 in 1960, falling to a low of in 2010 of 14.89 per 100,000. Over the decades during which the new generation of antidepressants, Medicare, and Medicaid were introduced and became widely used, suicide rates declined by a rate of nearly 10 deaths per 100,000 older Americans.

TABLE 8.1. Suicides in the United States among Persons Ages 65 and Older per 100,000 per Year across Six Decades

	1960	1970	1980	1990	2000	2010
Men and women	24.5	20.8	17.6	20.5	15.5	14.89
Men	44.0	38.4	35.0	41.6	30.9	29.40
Women	8.4	8.1	6.1	6.4	4.0	4.01
White men	46.7	41.1	37.2	44.2	34.5	31.9
Black men	9.9	8.7	11.4	14.9	11.2	9.85
White women	8.8	8.5	6.4	6.8	4.3	4.32
Black women		2.6		1.9	1.3	1.00
Hispanic men				23.4	17.2	15.27
Hispanic women					8.15[a]	2.28
Asian/Pacific men			18.6	16.8	18.1	15.44
Asian/Pacific women				8.5	5.7	4.81
American Indian/ Alaska Native					11.8[a]	3.96[a]
Total deaths			5,803[b]	6,394	5,306	5,858

Note. Data from 1980 on were retrieved July 17, 2012, from *webappa.cdc.gov/sasweb/ ncipc/mortrate10_us.html.*
[a] Considered unstable due to reported deaths less than 20.
[b] Data are from 1981.

However, the actual number of deaths (rather than the rates) approached the 1980 total in 2000 and surpassed it in 2010.

There were a total of 40,267,984 older Americans in 2010, making up more than 12% of the population. But they accounted for more than 15% of suicides. In 2010, there were 5,949 older adult suicides. Although the crude suicidal death rate was 14.89 per 100,000 seniors, including all races, ethnicities, and both genders, the highest suicide death rate observed was in white males ages 85 and above, at 50.82 per 100,000. The rate for white males ages 65 and above was 29 per 100,000. Suicide rates among males grow from late adolescence with an abrupt increase from age 65. From adolescence on, 70 percent of suicides occur among white males, climbing to more than 80 percent by age 85. In contrast, older women's suicide rates remain constant from age 65 (CDC, 2014). Although more women than men attempt suicide at all ages (Krug, 2004), older males commit suicide five times more often than older women. The preponderance of suicides among elderly white males, the population segment least likely to seek treatment for depression (Rutz et al., 1995), has been the case since the turn of the 20th century.

RISK OF SUICIDE AMONG OLDER ADULTS

The ratio of attempted suicide to suicidal death is 4:1 among older persons compared to 100:1 among those 15–24 years of age. This is partly explained by the differences in lethality of means chosen for the attempts. Of the nearly 6,000 suicides among older adults in 2010, more than 70% were the result of firearms. In 2005 there were 32,000 deaths due to suicide but more than 350,000 visits to emergency rooms and more than 150,000 hospital admissions due to suicidal and self-destructive behavior (McCaig & Nawar, 2006). Thus, while mortality from suicide can be said to account for only 5.7% of years of productive life lost population wide, the morbidity associated with attempted suicide is enormous.

In addition to advanced age and white race, state of residence is also related to suicide (see Figure 8.1). Of the 12 states with the highest prevalence of late-life suicide, 9 are in the West (CDC, 2014). These states also tend to be rural and sparsely populated, with less ease of access to one's neighbors, health care, and supportive services (Watts et al., 2007) and greater access to firearms (Miller, Azrael, & Barber, 2012). Among adults ages 55 and older who take their lives, 77% have seen their primary care provider within the past year and 58% within a month of their deaths. In contrast only 8.5% have received any form of mental health service within 1 year and 11% within one month. (Luoma, Martin, & Pearson, 2002). These statistics add to the profile of persons at risk of suicidal behavior, which is displayed in Table 8.2. The profile is useful for risk assessment among select populations such as depressed patients in clinical settings. But screening instruments to detect suicidal ideation generate too many false positives for universal application (Haney et al., 2012). For example, of 175 randomly selected older community residents who affirmed "thoughts that you would be better off dead or harming yourself" (see question 9 from the PHQ-9 in Figure 1.1) during a telephone interview with a nonclinician, only 70 indicated they had had suicidal ideas upon telephone follow-up with a psychiatrist (Kennedy et al., 2014).

The baby boomer generation born between 1946 and 1964 has already exhibited higher rates of suicide than those of their parents and

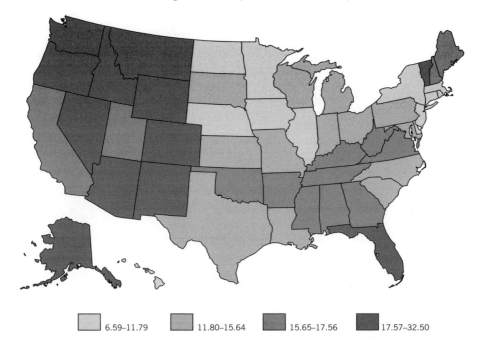

6.59–11.79 11.80–15.64 15.65–17.56 17.57–32.50

FIGURE 8.1. Death rates from injury and suicide in the United States among persons ages 64–85+ per 100,000, 2000–2006. Data from Centers for Disease Control and Prevention (2014). Web-based Injury Statistics Query and Reporting System (WISQARS). Available at *www.cdc.gov/ncipc/wisqars/default.htm*.

subsequent birth cohorts. The first of the baby boomers reached age 65 in 2011. The total number of older Americans is projected to be 71 million, or 20% of the U.S. population, by 2030 (CDC, 2007). In short, the cohort with historically elevated risk is about to enter the age range of additional elevated risk, doing so in large numbers. Thus both the rate and number of older adult suicides is expected to increase, reversing a trend sustained over the last 20 years (Conwell, Van Orden, & Caine, 2011).

Transmission and Persistence of Risk

A suicide attempt by a parent results in a sixfold increase in suicide attempts among his or her children (Brent et al., 2002). Therefore, the number of senior suicides, though comparatively small, imperils the subsequent generation. The cohort of middle-aged adults in the early 1980s

TABLE 8.2. Suicide Risk Profile

Historical
- Previous attempt
- Lethality of attempt: firearms, jumping
- Family history
- Low probability of rescue
- Recent visit to primary care physician or mental health specialist
- Anniversary of loss

Sociodemographic
- White male
- Age 85 years or older
- Firearms purchase, possession
- Divorced, widowed
- Recent life change event (hospitalization)

Clinical
- Expressed intent
- Depression or other nondementing mental disorder
- Alcohol use, moderate to heavy
- Cancer, heart disease, lung disease
- Chronic pain
- Poor self-assessed health
- Smoking

Note. Adapted from Kennedy (2000, p. 230). Copyright 2001 by The Guilford Press. Adapted by permission.

showed a higher rate of suicide than their grandparents (Haas & Hendin, 1983). The current prevalence of depression and suicide attempts at younger ages, coupled with the increasing number of older adults, suggests that the problem of late-life suicide will persist well into the 21st century (Conwell et al., 2011). In addition, there is little doubt that the actual number of suicides is underrepresented by suicide rates based on death certificates (Miller, 1978). And even though the numbers of assisted suicides remain small, they are increasing; increasing public acceptance of physician-assisted suicide, and by implication suicide in general, makes the concern all the more urgent (Finlay & George, 2011).

Pain, Cancer, and Chronic Illness as Risk Factors

Tang and Crane (2006) found the risk of suicidal death to be at least doubled in chronic pain patients. Twenty percent of persons with chronic pain reported suicidal ideation with 5–14% reporting a prior suicide attempt. Eight characteristics were associated with suicidality and chronic pain. These included initial insomnia as well as the type, intensity, and duration of pain. Also associated were the desire for escape from the pain, helplessness and hopelessness about pain, and catastrophic self-assessments. Deficits in problem-solving skills and an avoidant coping style were also prominent.

Many of these characteristics are targeted in cognitive-behavioral approaches to the prevention of suicide attempts (see Chapter 4 and Table 4.3). Brown et al. (2005) randomized 120 persons who had made a suicide attempt to cognitive therapy plus case management or case management alone. After 18 months participants who received cognitive therapy were half as likely to have reattempted suicide. They were significantly less depressed and hopeless despite having the same frequency of suicidal ideation as the comparison group. Nonetheless, 24% of those in cognitive therapy and 41% in case management made at least one subsequent suicide attempt. This study is a reminder that effective prevention is more often risk reduction than risk elimination.

Fang and associates (2012), conducted a historical cohort study examining the risk of suicide among persons recently diagnosed with cancer. Relative risk estimates were calculated from the week following diagnosis to more than a year afterward and compared to risk figures for cancer-free patients. The relative risk of suicide was increased tenfold for the cancer patients during the first week and threefold during the first year following the cancer diagnosis. Suicide rates were higher among patients with preexisting psychiatric diagnoses whether or not they had received a recent diagnosis of cancer. However, relative risks of suicide following a cancer diagnosis were higher among persons without a preexisting mental disorder. As expected, the rates and relative risks of suicide among men exceeded those among women regardless of diagnosis. The relative risk of suicide among those with a cancer diagnosis did not differ by age, with the exception of the 65- to 74-year age group, whose relative risk was nearly four times higher than that for other groups.

This study is all the more noteworthy for the sample size, range of cancers included, unequivocal outcomes, and comparison of two causes of death, cancer and suicide, that share behavioral risk factors, namely, smoking and excessive alcohol intake. Because risk of death was most elevated in the 7 days after the diagnosis, the emotional impact of having cancer rather than the progression of the disease seems more likely to be driving the phenomenon. In addition, the authors did not investigate other outcomes such as nonfatal hospitalization due to suicide attempts or mental illness. As a result, their findings likely underestimate the risk of suicidal behavior from receiving a diagnosis of cancer.

Cancer is not the only illness associated with an elevated risk of suicide. In an 8-year study of nearly 600 family medicine practices in the United Kingdom, Webb et al. (2012) matched patients with one of 11 specific diagnoses by age and gender to patients without any of the identified conditions. Relative risk estimates of death were made possible by linkage to the national mortality records. The authors sought to identify diagnoses reported to increase the risk of suicide and to determine the extent to which depression, gender, and advanced age might contribute to risk. Conditions examined included cancer, coronary heart disease, hypertension, stroke, diabetes, asthma, chronic obstructive pulmonary disease (COPD), osteoarthritis, osteoporosis, back pain, and epilepsy. Patients were classified as depressed if any current or past episode of depressive disorder was recorded unless coded as "remitted" at the time of death. Age matching precluded the potential confounding effect of youth.

Among men and women combined, relative risk of suicide was elevated in association with four conditions: coronary heart disease, stroke, COPD, and osteoporosis, with mean ages of 74, 79, 66, and 77, respectively. The size of risk ranged from 50% greater for coronary heart disease to more than twofold for osteoporosis. However, when adjusted for the presence of depression, risk estimates declined considerably but remained significantly elevated for these four conditions. Among women the relative risk of suicide increased significantly and substantially as the number of co-occurring diagnoses mounted. Women with three or more diagnoses experienced a greater than twofold increase in the odds of suicide; they had a mean age of 77 years. Among women, the relative risk of suicide was significantly and substantially elevated for cancer and coronary heart disease with a nearly twofold elevation in risk remaining after adjusting for depression. The authors concluded that among older women, depression did not explain the association of suicide with cancer or coronary heart disease. They questioned the hypothesis that physical illness leads to suicide through depression but were unable to explore the potential contribution of disability.

Modifiable Suicide Risk Factors

The search for modifiable suicide risk factors has focused on suicidal ideas among younger community residents, select clinical samples of older patients from primary care and psychiatric settings, or postmortem examinations of suicidal deaths. In these studies, depression is the predominant but not the sole predictor of suicide. Data from clinical studies indicate that a depressive episode has been experienced by two-thirds or more of older adults who commit suicide (Conwell, Duberstein, & Caine, 2002). However, in Conwell and colleagues' psychological autopsy study nearly a quarter of the sample appeared to be free of diagnosable psychopathology (Conwell et al., 1991). Fifty-four percent of those in the sample had been diagnosed with a major depressive disorder, 11% with minor depression. Of note, only 68% of coroner-identified cases had collateral informants willing and able to provide information for the study.

Population attributable risk estimates the percentage of suicides that might be reduced by removal of a specific risk factor such as depression. Beautrais et al. (2002) estimated that ameliorating the risk factor of diminished social networks of some older adults would reduce suicide in the population (i.e., population attributable risk) by 27%. Elimination of depressive symptoms would reduce the prevalence of suicidal ideation by less than 50%. Elimination of traumatic events would reduce suicides by slightly more than a third (Goldney et al., 2000). Similarly, Cavanagh et al.'s 2003 systematic review of 76 psychological autopsy studies found from one-quarter to one-half of the population attributable risk for suicide was due to psychosocial factors other than mental illness.

The case fatality ratio (CFR) is another useful statistic with substantial implications for prevention. The CFR for suicide is the number of deaths divided by the number of attempts. The use of a highly lethal method such has suffocation or firearms elevates the CFR. In the United States differences in both the geographic and demographic distribution of the CFR for suicide are predominantly explained by firearms (Miller et al., 2012). However, until the 2012 murder of schoolchildren and their teachers in Newtown, Connecticut, the relationship between firearms and suicide received little attention (*New York Times*, 2013). The population attributable risk for suicide among older adults due to guns is better than 70%. Clearly the elimination of firearms in the United States is unrealistic, but given the high associated CFR, a modest reduction in self-inflicted gunshots would have obvious benefits. Several states have opted to focus on "gun safety," rather than the more inflammatory term "gun control," by advocating for trigger locks or lock boxes in the home to keep lethal means out of the hands of impulsive, mentally ill family members (Tavernise, 2013).

The concepts of population attributable risk and CFR are clearly useful, but they do not address countervailing forces, that is, reasons to live. Table 8.3 lists some that, if present, might mitigate risk, and if they are present but not optimal, they might be enhanced though environmental, social, or behavioral interventions.

COLLABORATIVE CARE, SSRIs, AND SUICIDE PREVENTION IN PRIMARY CARE

Since the advent of the SSRIs, as noted above, many more antidepressants have been prescribed, but the reduction in suicides has been relatively slight. A population-based study of Ontario residents ages 65 and older (Mamdani, Herrman, & Austin, 1999) found an increase in antidepressant prescriptions. The highest antidepressant utilization rates were observed for women ages 85–89, with more than 17% receiving an antidepressant by 1997. Carlsten et al. (2001) found a similar increase in antidepressant utilization with the introduction of the SSRIs between 1977 and 1997 in Sweden with highest rates noted among seniors. This was accompanied by a significant decline in the slope of suicide rates among both men and women, with half the number of "saved lives" occurring among young adults. However, Barbui et al. (1999) found little change in overall suicide rates across Italy between 1966 and 1988 despite an increase in the sales of SSRIs. The modest decline in suicides among women was countered by an increase among men.

TABLE 8.3. Countervailing Forces (Reasons to Live) That Might Lessen the Older Adult's Likelihood of Acting on a Suicidal Impulse

- Satisfaction with social support
- Presence of spouse or partner
- Social network
- Financial security
- Physical independence or autonomously stable dependency
- Alcohol abstinence
- Dementia (inability to sequence steps toward death)
- Positively anticipated life events of family members
- Religious beliefs and values (optimistic rather than fatalistic)
- Advance directives, health care proxy
- Practitioner's optimism and concern, regular appointments for ongoing care
- Engaged in treatment of depression, anxiety, insomnia, pain

Note. Adapted from Plutchik et al. (1996). Copyright 1996 by John Wiley & Sons, Inc. Adapted by permission.

Ganguli et al. (1997) found only 5% of a population of 1,681 seniors in southwestern Pennsylvania used an antidepressant during four waves of interviews between 1987 and 1996 despite a substantial change from tricyclics to SSRIs. Steffens et al. (2000), reporting on the Cache Country survey of more than 4,500 older community residents, found that two-thirds of those with major depression did not receive an antidepressant. Unützer (2006) reported a marked increase in antidepressant treatment among the "routine care" arm of the IMPACT study, which integrates a "depression specialist" to aggressively treat depression in the randomized intervention group. However, despite the increase in antidepressant prescriptions the severity of depression changed little if at all. Even when antidepressants achieve a remission of symptoms, recurrence rates are likely to be higher among those patients with suicidal ideas. Szanto et al. (2001) found equivalent remission rates between depressed elders with suicidal ideas (77%) and those without (78%). However, the relapse rate doubled (26% vs. 13%) when suicidal ideas were reported.

After the introduction of SSRIs, antidepressant prescriptions increased by 400% in the United States, but over the same period suicidal deaths declined by only 3% (Mann et al., 2005). The substitution of SSRIs, which are rarely lethal in overdose, for tricyclic antidepressants, which are highly lethal in overdose, may be responsible for the decline. Although antidepressant prescriptions provided by primary care physicians have increased, the number of psychotherapy visits has declined. Moreover, the largest increase in antidepressants has been among young adults, children, and adolescents (McKeown, Cuffe, & Schulz, 2006). These facts further support the findings, reviewed in Chapter 5, that initial treatment with an antidepressant alone is often insufficient for reducing depression. Aggressive treatment using collaborative care models can reduce late-life depression, but can they also reduce suicidal behaviors?

The IMPACT study mentioned above and the PROSPECT study (Skultety & Zeiss, 2006; Woltman et al., 2012), which attempted to reduce suicidality as well as depression, are examined in greater detail next. IMPACT and PROSPECT were both examples of collaborative chronic care models (see Chapter 9, Table 9.2) and shared a common method of integrating nurses into primary care sites as depression managers to improve the outcome of depression treatment.

PROSPECT

The PROSPECT study employed a two-step screening procedure (Bruce et al., 2004; Alexopoulos et al., 2009). Persons with a clinically significant level of depressive symptoms assessed by telephone were sub-sequently administered an in-person structured diagnostic interview and the Beck Scale for Suicidal Ideation (Beck, Kovacs, & Weissman, 1979). Twelve percent of those screened (599 persons), mostly women (71%), reported a significant level of depressive symptoms, two-thirds with major, one-third with minor depression.

Nearly 90% of collaborative care patients received either antide-pressant medication, psychotherapy, or both, in contrast to 49–62% of routine care patients. Among participants with major depression at baseline, 35% of collaborative care and 24% of routine care patients reported suicidal ideation. However, by month 4, the rates were nearly equivalent at 20% versus 19%, respectively, but the decline within the collaborative care group was statistically significant. The differences were also significant at months 8 and 24 but not at months 12 and 18. At 24 months, 11% of collaborative care and 15% of routine care patients continued to express suicidal ideation, but the overall decline in suicidal ideation was 3.2 times greater among the collaborative care group. In contrast, among persons with minor depression there were no significant differences detected between the two groups at any time. At baseline, 14% of collaborative care and 9% of routine care patients expressed suicidal ideation, declining to 11% and 6% by 24 months, respectively.

Depression treatment response was defined by a 50% reduction in symptom severity measured with the HAM-D. The collaborative care group experienced a significant response at each evaluation throughout 24 months. Between months 18 and 24 there was a 9% increase in the percentage responding to the collaborative care intervention in contrast to a 3% decline among routine care patients with major depression. Ulti-mately 64% of collaborative care patients versus 40% of routine care patients had responded. For intervention patients, the remission rates went from 27% at 4 months to 45% at 24 months, compared to 15% and 32% for routine care. For persons with minor depression, remis-sion rates went from slightly above 40% to 60% at 24 months with no significant differences observed between intervention and routine care. Stated differently, the majority of collaborative care patients with major depression were better, but most were not well, and 10% continued to express suicidal ideas. Among persons receiving routine care, most were not better, only a third were well, and 15% continued to have suicidal ideas. Among those with minor depression at baseline, most were well at 24 months, but suicidal thinking remained among 6–12%.

IMPACT

In the IMPACT study, 13.3% of depressed primary care patients randomized to routine care and 15.9% in the collaborative care group expressed thoughts of suicide. Patients in the collaborative care intervention group exhibited significantly lower rates of active suicidal ideation at 6 months (7.5% vs. 12.1%) and at 12 months (9.8% vs. 15.5%). After depression care managers were withdrawn, active ideation remained significantly lower among the intervention group at 18 months (8.0% vs. 13.3%) and 24 months (10.1% vs. 13.9%). The intervention was also significantly more effective than routine care in reducing passive thoughts of death at 6 months (27% vs. 38%), 13 months (32% vs. 51%), 18 months (38% vs. 50%), and 24 months (41% vs. 50%). Passive thoughts of death are not necessarily suicidal in the context of life-threatening illness and old age. In addition, significantly more patients in routine care received an emergency evaluation because of suicidal impulses than did those in the intervention group (7.7% vs. 4.3%) (Unützer et al., 2006).

Passive versus Active Thoughts of Suicide

There is controversy over the extent to which passive thoughts of death as assessed in PROSPECT and IMPACT predict risk of active suicidal ideation (Raue et al., 2006). Passive thoughts of death such as "weak desire to live today," the first item from the Scale for Suicidal Ideation (Beck et al., 1979) or "Thoughts that you would be better off dead, or of hurting yourself in some way," the ninth item from the PHQ-9 (Kroenke & Spitzer, 2002), do not include suicide. Because thoughts of death may represent a realistic appraisal in the context of life-threatening illness or extreme old age, care must be taken to distinguish death ideation from suicidal thought. But to what extent do passive thoughts of death relate to explicit thoughts of suicide?

The PROSPECT study defined patients with a "weak desire to live today" as having suicidal ideas. This threshold was purposefully chosen in light of Brown et al.'s (2005) finding that psychiatric patients ages 55 and older with "weak desire to live today" exhibited a risk of suicide 15.5 times higher than those who did not. Walker and associates (2010b) performed follow-up telephone interviews of 330 patients enrolled as outpatients in a cancer center who acknowledged they had had "thoughts you might be better off dead or harming yourself in some way" in the last 2 weeks as documented by completion of the PHQ-9. One-third of the group denied those thoughts and one-third acknowledged them but denied suicidal ideation. The remaining third reported explicit thoughts of suicide. Persons who indicated they had "thoughts you might be better off dead or harming yourself in some way" more than half the days in the last 2 weeks were more likely to express explicit suicidal ideation. However, 23% of those (54 out of 235) who confirmed the thoughts had occurred for "several days," and as a result scored only 1 on the ninth PHQ-9 item, were also found to have suicidal thoughts (Walker et al., 2010a).

In a study of patients being treated for recurrent depressive disorders, Szanto et al. (1996) found that those with passive suicidal thoughts who denied intent to harm themselves were as pessimistic about the future as those with active suicidal thoughts. As treatment continued, active suicidal thoughts became passive before disappearing entirely, suggesting a continuum of risk.

In summary, most older persons with passive thoughts of death will not acknowledge thoughts of suicide. But reaching the minority who do justifies the additional effort of asking about suicide. More specifically, the ninth item from the PHQ-9 should not be omitted to reduce the false positive rate of suicidal ideation when screening clinical populations. It may well represent the patient's relative status on a continuum of suicidal risk. However, when clinicians communicate concerns to one another, it is preferable to quote the patient's exact words rather than characterize them as "passive thoughts of suicide." Table 1.4 offered practitioner guidelines for assessing suicide risk in patients who express thoughts of death or suicide.

In summary, both the PROSPECT and IMPACT studies integrated specially trained mental health personnel into primary care settings. Both studies monitored adherence to antidepressant guidelines and provided guidance to physicians and patients when deviations occurred. Both psychotherapy and psychiatric consultations were readily available. However, both depressive symptoms and suicidal ideas remained in a minority of patients in both studies despite their interventions. These studies demonstrate the extent to which suicidality may be reduced when the effort is purely clinic based.

REDUCING SUICIDALITY BEYOND PRIMARY CARE

Using population-based studies of cardiovascular disease risk factor identification, Knox et al. (2004) argued that we lack a genuine epidemiology of suicidal risk other than clinically identified high-risk elements such as major depression or prior suicide attempts. It is unlikely that the reductions in cardiovascular deaths could have been realized without investigating the role of dietary fat as well as angina in the development of myocardial infarction. Citing the Air Force Suicide Prevention Program, Knox, Conwell, and Caine (2003) demonstrated how a systematic intervention outside the clinical arena aimed at changing social norms about help seeking can have substantial impact.

Paykel et al.'s (1997) Defeat Depression Campaign included public information efforts to reduce stigma and promote treatment as well as to update physicians on advances in diagnosis and treatment of depression. Suicide rates declined by 11.7%. A similar public education effort in Australia titled "beyondblue" resulted in an increase in public awareness (Jorm, Christensen, & Griffiths, 2005). Suicide rates were reduced and antidepressant prescriptions increased on the island of Gotland, Sweden, through an intensive educational program for primary care physicians (Rutz et al., 1995). However, none of these programs employed a comparison population, and the observed effects may have been due to events not associated with the intervention.

While and colleagues (2012) provide evidence that incorporating recommendations into clinical settings is related to reduction in suicidal deaths. Several recommendations, such as assertive community outreach to patients not adhering to treatment, were associated with reduced deaths over a 10-year period ending in 2006. Mental health programs that incorporated more recommendations exhibited greater reductions in suicides. Although the study included mental health clinics only and thereby a smaller population at identified risk of suicide rather than the larger universal population, it demonstrated that interventions are effective if implemented in broad-based, systematic fashion.

Mann et al.'s (2005) comprehensive review of strategies for preventing suicide across all age groups identified the following health and social policies: (1) awareness and education, including physician education and gatekeeper training; (2) screening; (3) treatment interventions; (4) means restriction (e.g., bridges, firearms); and (5) codes of conduct for media coverage. However, only screening and treatment interventions have been examined in relation to older adult suicide (Lapierre et al., 2011). Of the 19 studies that focused on older adults, the approaches included primary care intervention, community-based outreach, telephone counseling, or clinical treatment, meaning psychiatric specialty care or therapeutic groups based on either cognitive-behavioral or interpersonal psychotherapy. Most programs addressed risks and reliably reduced symptoms of depression and ideas of suicide. However, there was little or no effect on males. Two programs that attempted to improve protective factors in small psychotherapeutic groups were associated with significant and persistent reduction in suicidal ideation and depression; the protective factors included behavioral activation, increased resiliency, improved pursuit of personal goals (Lapierre et al., 2007), and enhanced social support (Heisel et al., 2009).

None of the prevention programs addressed substance use in older men, even though a retrospective case–control study showed that alcohol dependence or misuse was observed in 35% of the older males who died by suicide (Waern, 2003). Alcohol use disorder remained an independent predictor of suicide risk. In addition, several studies found that sleep disturbances or painful chronic diseases were associated with suicidal ideation. Other characteristics, such as forced retirement, bereavement, diminished self-reliance, and loss of one's driver's license, may provide more effective avenues to reach males disinclined to speak of depression, alcohol abuse, or loss of self-esteem.

The Nuremberg Alliance against Depression

The Nuremberg Alliance against Depression (NAD) to reduce suicidality was a study using a multilevel intervention to compare suicidal deaths and suicide attempts over 2 years in Nuremberg and Würzburg, Germany. As shown in Table 8.4, a comprehensive community and clinical intervention consisting of four levels was directed at the population of Nuremberg. Würzburg received observation only. The four levels of intervention were designed to saturate the environment with a social marketing campaign to recognize and reduce depression and thereby suicidality. The campaign was focused on primary care physicians, patients, and their families, and also incorporated communications media as well as facilitators to serve as case sentinels and informal community advisers. At both 12 and 24 months following the intervention, rates of suicide declined in both cities, although the reductions were statistically significant in neither. However, the decline in suicide attempts was significantly and substantially greater from baseline to 12 months (–18.3%) and 24 months (*Note.* 26.5%) in Nuremberg but not in Würzburg. The reductions in attempts were most noticeable for highly lethal means (shooting, hanging, and jumping) and among persons less than 70 years of age (Hegerl et al., 2006).

TABLE 8.4. The Nuremberg Alliance against Depression: Four Levels of Intervention

- Primary care physicians
  - o Interactive educational sessions with videotape and guideline-driven antidepressant prescribing
  - o Single-page laminated screening, diagnosis, and treatment guide
  - o Educational videotape for patients and family members
  - o Specialist hotline for individualized advice to the physician
- The media, other professionals, and the community
  - o Reportage guidelines to newspapers, television, and radio to prevent imitation suicides
  - o Publicity campaign to destigmatize depression
  - o Movie trailers, posters, brochures, lectures, website
  - o Politicians enlisted as patrons of the campaign
- Community facilitators
  - o 2,000 priests, teachers, policemen, pharmacists, prison officers, helpline workers, counseling center staff, psychotherapists, primary care professionals, geriatric caregivers
  - o Training in depression recognition and advice giving
- Patients and their families
  - o Peer support groups
  - o EZ pass access card to specialists for suicide attempters

Note. Based on Hegerl et al. (2006).

The Oregon Older Adult Suicide Prevention Plan

Similar to the Nuremberg Alliance, the Oregon Older Adult Suicide Prevention Plan involved the broadest possible attack on the elements of suicidal risk in late life. Plan development funds were provided by Oregon's Office of Disease Prevention and Epidemiology, but subsequent implementation funds have been made available for youth suicide prevention and not specifically for older adults. Nonetheless, collaboration between Oregon's Senior Disability Services program and the Youth Suicide Prevention initiative has assisted 19 counties to increase the number of persons trained to intervene. The interventions use the Question, Persuade, Refer (*www.qprinstitute.com*) method and Applied Suicide Intervention Skills Training (ASIST; *www.livingworks.net*), which are applicable to the needs of older adults as well as youth (D. Noonan, personal communication, August 15, 2012). Table 8.5 is a reduced list of the strategic objectives for Oregon's clinical, community-based, and public health interventions for older adults. The introduction of integrated models of depression care into primary practice is but one element of the program. The hoped-for broad implementation of the initiative has not been

TABLE 8.5. Oregon's Suicide Prevention Strategies for Older Adults

Strategy 1: Prevention in the clinical venue

- Objective 1.0 Primary care
  o Improve screening, assessment, and risk reduction among primary care providers
  o Increase educational content regarding late-life depression and suicide for the health professions at graduate and postgraduate levels including licensing, certification, and maintenance of certification
  o Implement integrated models of behavioral health and primary care
  o Streamline, expedite referral systems and patterns

- Objective 1.1 Workforce
  o Increase the supply of specialists in geriatrics

- Objective 1.2 Financing
  o Increase funds for both primary care and behavioral health specialists
  o Parity for behavioral health services within primary care insurance plans

- Objective 1.3 Outreach
  o Telephone-facilitated care links for rural areas
  o Recruit home care agency nurses and parish nurses for screening
  o Extend services to rural areas, integrate behavioral health, primary care, and social service agencies including those serving Native Americans

Strategy 2: Community-based prevention

- Objective 2.0 Develop incentives, procedures for state and local partnerships
  o Mobilize local coalitions of older adults, both new and existing
  o Activate statewide government agencies and offices, commissions, associations, businesses, communities of faith
  o Coordinate county mental health plans with the private sector for improved implementation and evaluation strategies
  o Capture new resources through governmental and nonprofit entities and foundations

- Objective 2.1 Attack prejudicial attitudes regarding aging, mental illness and mental health care, and the presumed inevitability of suicide with a coordinated campaign of education and social marketing
  o Create broadly based educational materials for the widest possible audience
  o Reach out to the public, the professions, legislators, policy makers, social, fraternal, and faith-based groups, middle school, high school, colleges

- Objective 2.2 Improve formal case reporting procedures and the media's approach to suicide and mental illness
  o Disseminate guidelines for case reports to mental health professionals, community advocates, and service agencies
  o Promulgate media reportage guidelines
  o Create media watchdog groups to monitor reportage

- Objective 2.3 Train community members in intervention skills
  o Develop a cadre of trainers for professionals, first responders, and community residents
  o Offer ongoing technical assistance to the trainers

(continued)

TABLE 8.5. *(continued)*

- Objective 2.4 Increase perceived social support, reduce isolation
  - Advertise the value of social cohesion
  - Reach out to isolated seniors
  - Institute telephone support and crisis line services
  - Encourage the use of bereavement support groups and peer counselors

- Objective 2.5 Enhance coping skills and opportunities
  - Improve access to home care, rehabilitation, pain management, palliative care services
  - Reorient health care and social services to reduce disability and promote autonomy as well as the management of chronic disease

- Objective 2.6 Minimize access to lethal means
  - Implement safer prescribing practices and dispensing procedures
  - Train health and social service providers to inquire about lethal means
  - Ally with the Oregon Gun Owners Association
  - Educate the public about lethal means and measures to reduce their availability

- Objective 2.7 Undermine negative stereotypes about aging
  - Encourage journalists to portray older adults as a resource rather than a burden
  - Educate youth groups about the resilience, wisdom, and other positive aspects of aging
  - Advertise senior mentors and role models

- Objective 2.8 Create policies to enhance seniors' social engagement
  - Reduce age discrimination
  - Assemble a task force to identify elements of a more senior-friendly environment and means of transportation

Srategy 3: Surveillance, evaluation, and research

- Objective 3.0 Improve public health surveillance systems and reporting procedures to generate greater detail on suicidality in late life
  - Upgrade or implement the Violent Death Reporting System, Behavioral Risk Factor Surveillance System, Adolescent Suicide Attempts Data System
  - Quality improvement of existing systems

- Objective 3.1 Encourage preventative intervention evaluations
  - Provide technical assistance to increase the number of interventions with evaluation components
  - Publish, disseminate outcomes

- Objective 3.2 Expand the base for scientific research
  - Create a statewide research agenda
  - Establish a network of scientists focused on suicide prevention

Note. Adapted from the Oregon Older Adult Suicide Prevention Plan (retrieved August 10, 2012, from *http://egov.oregon.gov/DHS/ph/ipe/esp/docs/plan.pdf*).

completed. Yet the evidence supporting the integration of depression care managers into primary care is among the strongest to date.

Suicide Prevention in Adult Retirement Communities

In 2008 the U.S. Substance Abuse and Mental Health Services Administration (SAMHSA) funded the development by the National Association of State Mental Health Program Directors (NASMHPD) of a suicide prevention toolkit for residents of senior living communities (SLCs), including nursing homes and assisted living, independent living, and continuing care retirement communities. The SPARK (Suicide Prevention Assessment and Resource Kit) toolkit, Promoting Emotional Health and Preventing Suicide: A Toolkit for Senior Living Communities, is available at *http://store.samhsa.gov/product/SMA10-4515*. NASMHPD subcontracted with three organizations—the Education Development Center, Inc., McFarland Associates, and the NASMHPD Research Institute—to develop and evaluate the toolkit. Podgorski et al. (2010) summarized the background of the project and the recommendations that emerged. First, they noted that many of the underlying events that lead older adults to relocate to an SLC are stressful and complicate the adjustment to new surroundings, neighbors, and norms. These events include increased physical vulnerability, illness, and loss of spouse or caregiver. Although increased opportunities for socialization, support, and activity foster resilience and adaptation to loss, they may be accompanied by a "frailty identity crisis" (Fillit & Butler, 2009) in which absolute independence is sacrificed for sustainable interdependence. Furthermore, cognitive impairment affects more than half the residents of nursing homes and assisted living facilities. One can argue that these facilities are mental health residences, yet the staffing, structure, and activity pattern are meant to promote a home-like atmosphere rather than treat or prevent mental illness. Although suicide is rare in these facilities, the impact of an attempt is devastating to residents, their families, and the staff.

Podgorski et al. (2010) recommend a number of ways to reduce the risk of suicide in residential settings, which must be adapted to the culture and resources of each facility. First, for those residents at identified risk a variety of steps to reduce barriers to care should be adopted. These include stigma reduction programs and education about interventions to enhance help-seeking behaviors. Gatekeeper training should be provided to clinical staff, residents, and families to better identify and refer distressed individuals for help. This also entails screening for substance abuse, depression, and suicidal ideation. The profile of characteristics associated with depressive symptoms among residents of assisted living facilities includes greater disability, negative attitudes toward aging, poorer self-rated health, less sense of mastery, and less religiosity.

Screening must be linked with mental health services, ideally from on-site providers. This includes use of care management models for depression and substance abuse as well as increased monitoring of residents at identified risk. Pain and medical conditions causing multimorbidity and polypharmacy should be addressed with guideline-directed care, consultation, and interventions for specific disabilities.

A universal approach for all residents focuses on the promotion of coping and improved function through problem solving with an emphasis on role transitions, bereavement, and financial advice. Social networking among residents and families is encouraged to foster a sense of community and connectedness. This includes ready access to spiritual and religious activities, recreation, volunteering, and exercise. Finally, the facility needs to restrict access to firearms, stored chemicals, and prescriptions, to lessen the size of windows, and prohibit access to or create barriers to jumping from the roof.

REACHING MALES

Conwell (2009) illuminates the mixed blessing of the current status of suicide prevention research. With one exception, the reductions in suicidal ideation have been achieved among women, not men. With the majority of completed suicides occurring in men, the promise of these interventions remains unfulfilled. Focusing on depression yields clear benefits both in primary care and in community-based interventions such as the Nuremberg Alliance against Depression. The population attributable risk for suicide associated with depression is substantial. Nonetheless, the positive predictive value of depression as a risk factor for suicidal behavior is low. Few depressed people ever attempt suicide. Similarly, hopelessness and suicidal ideation are strongly associated with suicidal acts but are neither necessary nor sufficient to predict the majority of suicides (Batterham & Christensen, 2012). Reducing the morbidity of suicidal ideation and suicide attempts reduces individual suffering and the social burden. Yet the task of engaging men, who may perceive thoughts of death as a late-life norm rather than a manifestation of a treatable depressive illness, remains elusive. Because older, suicidal males are more likely to be socially disconnected (Conwell & Thompson, 2008), there may be little in the way of friends, family, or peers to leverage interventions for their benefit.

INSIGHTS FROM THE ARMED SERVICES

Although suicides among active-duty and discharged United States military personnel occur predominantly before old age, the current epidemic of suicidal deaths provides insights into the difficulty of suicide prevention as well as the extent of effort needed to effect change. Similar to suicide in late life, the majority of suicides by military personnel occur among white males, and predominantly with firearms. Warner et al. (2011) described a program of predeployment screening to indicate service personnel deemed too vulnerable for deployment and select those in need of additional interventions prior to deployment to Iraq. Subsequent contacts for suicidal ideation, combat-related stress, and psychiatric disorders, as well as occupational impairment and evacuation due to behavioral problems, were all less among the brigades that were subject to screening. In addition to screening, postdeployment services were coordinated with primary care providers to ensure continuity, sustain confidentiality, and avoid the stigma of referral to a mental health specialist. Efforts to provide systems-level collaborative care for depression and PTSD understandably lagged behind the need as the ramp-up to war was not accompanied by a similarly rapid preparation for its aftermath (Engel et al., 2008).

Despite the measures described above, suicide rates have continued to increase and have received attention by both civilian policy makers and general staff. Among active-duty personnel, deaths due to suicide have exceeded those due to combat, leading Hoge and Castro (2012) to argue for the need for programs that far exceed screening and risk assessment, including education to create public awareness of suicide, similar to that for other life-threatening conditions. Treatment approaches must include enhanced access, sustained engagement, and coordinated care. The protective effects of family and peer relations should be reinforced, and access to lethal means should be restricted. To prevent recurrent attempts, evidence-based psychosocial interventions such as PST, DBT, and CBT should be employed.

Katz (2012) echoes the call for public education and reinforcement of social cohesion, arguing that suicides among veterans began to decline as the public became more aware of the realities of postdeployment stress, a phenomenon he calls "the yellow ribbon effect." Caine (2012) calls for a new coalition of advocacy groups to organize for more broadly based policies for research as well as reduction in deaths due to suicide and all forms of interpersonal violence. These would include persons with a family member who died by suicide or homicide as well as victims of intimate partner violence. He also calls for a greater awareness of socially important "pre-suicidal" conditions. His assertion that the Department of Veterans Affairs and the Department of Defense will have much to teach seems particularly apt for the enduring problem of suicide among older males. Even with the best of intentions, senior leadership, and interventions across an array of venues, the tragedy of military suicide remains far too frequent.

CONCLUSION

The technology of depression care has advanced substantially, with important implications for the reduction of suicidality in late life. Yet lessons emerging from efforts to reduce suicides among veterans and active-duty military personnel underscore the need for a much broader approach similar to, but farther-reaching than the Nuremberg Alliance against Depression. One can argue that the universal health care available to residents of Germany and to U.S. armed forces and veterans offers an example of how preventive interventions might be coordinated and how health policy can be forged expeditiously when public support is mobilized. The notion that psychopathology and social pathology are competing rather than complementary opportunities for intervention has ceased to be reasonable. Suicide prevention best exemplifies the need to move from clinic-based to population-based approaches to mental health, approaches that are both collaborative and comprehensive, with sufficient evidence of benefits to justify implementation (U.S. Department of Health and Human Services, Office of the Surgeon General, and National Action Alliance for Suicide Prevention, 2012).

CHAPTER 9

Prevention of Depression: Implications for Collaborative Care

Worldwide mental illness is the leading cause of years of life lost to disability. Depressive disorders account for 40% of that figure, outstripping both the psychoses and substance abuse disorders (Whiteford et al., 2013). Without major changes in the allocation of health resources the disability associated with depression will persist or grow (Patel & Shekar, 2014) for several reasons. At best, only 50% of patients with major depression respond fully to initial antidepressant treatment. An additional third will recover if the antidepressant is switched to another agent or augmented with a second antidepressant or psychotherapy. For those who do recover, 40–60% will experience recurrence. A significant minority will experience recurrence due to premature cessation of treatment.

A confluence of factors suggests that prevention strategies must be added to treatment protocols if the burden of depressive illness is to be substantially reduced. Although disease prevention has immense public appeal, perceived benefits of preventive interventions must justify their inevitable burdens, more so when the intervention is contaminated with the stigma of mental illness. With the advent of collaborative care models of mental health services (see Table 9.2) and the passage of the Mental Health Parity and Addiction Equity Act, reducing the incidence of depression among older adults seems possible. This chapter discusses the avenues and obstacles to the prevention of depression, the confusing terminology, to highlight the challenge of preventing depression.

THE DISEASE BURDEN OF DEPRESSION

We measure *mortality* in years of life lost (YLL) to premature death. The leading causes of mortality are diseases with high fatality rates. Included among those diseases are ischemic heart disease and cerebrovascular disease, accounting for 25% of all deaths in higher-income nations. In contrast, unipolar depression, adult-onset hearing loss, and alcohol use disorders are the leading causes of healthy years lost to *disability*, accounting for 25% of the total. Clearly, depression after age 60 is a pressing concern. Depression frequently occurs with impaired vision, heart attack, stroke, and dementia and amplifies the disability associated with them.

THE CHALLENGE OF RISK IDENTIFICATION FOR DEPRESSION

A true indicator of risk predicts who is likely to become ill or disabled. However, the prediction of risk is relative rather than absolute. Most often, risk factors are neither completely necessary nor fully sufficient to produce illness. Some ill individuals will never have been exposed to the risk; some of those exposed will never develop the illness. Not all indicators of risk have direct preventive potential.

A *fixed indicator* is not changeable and thus not a target of intervention, although it may circumscribe the vulnerable population, as is the case with white males and suicide.

A *variable indicator,* such as age, might change spontaneously or through intervention, as with body weight, alcohol intake, or cigarette smoking. Variable risk indicators that cannot be modified (or have no discernable impact on the emergence of a disorder when modified) are called *variable risk markers*. Markers are important because they allow the potential population for prevention to be narrowed without specifying what the intervention should be. A variable indicator is considered a *causal risk factor* if the association is substantial or if an intervention targeting the indicator is proven to lessen the incidence of the disorder.

For example, the epidemiological association between cigarette smoking and lung cancer was so strong that it was considered causal. The reduction in lung cancer associated with smoking reduction provided further proof of causality. Even a true indicator of risk may not be causal and may itself be a proxy for an unappreciated psychosocial, biomedical, or disease-causing agent.

Examples Specific to Depression

Bereavement in late life is a fixed marker for the incidence of depression. However, the self-imposed social withdrawal that may follow bereavement is a changeable behavior. As described in Chapter 4, interventions to help the bereaved person sustain a rhythm of social engagement reduce the incidence of depression in late life (Prigerson et al., 1995/1996). Thus it is the loss of social rhythms that is a causal risk factor for depression, and not bereavement itself.

Another causal risk factor for depression is high-dose interferon-alpha therapy for melanoma (Musselman et al., 2001). High-dose interferon-alpha predictably triggers a major depressive disorder in 25% of treated individuals. However, major depression can be prevented in the majority of patients being treated with interferon-alpha through the use of prophylactic antidepressant treatment. More important, such prophylactic treatment significantly reduces the number of persons terminating interferon treatment due to adverse reactions.

Another population with an elevated prevalence of depressive disorders is persons with age-related macular degeneration. In a randomized trial, Rovner and Casten (2008) found a substantial reduction in the incidence of major depression and withdrawal from favored activities among older patients who received PST compared to those who received routine care and depression assessments only. Persons with a diagnosis of macular degeneration in one eye were approached for study participation at the time of diagnosis of macular degeneration in the second eye. Those randomized to PST received six 45- to 60-minute in-home sessions over 8 weeks. At 8 weeks 23.6% of those in routine care met diagnostic criteria for major depression compared to 11.2% of the intervention group. Six months later, 27.4% of those in routine care exhibited major depression compared to 21.1% of the intervention group—but the differences were no longer significant. However, the difference in percentage that had abandoned a valued activity was significant at both 2 and 6 months, with nearly twice the percentage of routine care participants reporting a loss. Analyses of mediating variables found PST prevented depression by lessening the abandonment of valued activities.

Although the groups were nearly free of depressive symptoms at the outset of the study, those who reported depressed mood were more likely to develop a depressive disorder. Presence of any level of depressed mood increased the risk of developing a depressive disorder 16-fold. Presence of insomnia doubled the risk. Although the preventive effect of PST on depressed mood was limited to the 2-month intervention, the reduction in disability carried over to 6 months, and fewer than 1 in 10 patients declined to complete the 8-week intervention. The number of patients one would need to treat with PST to prevent one episode of major depression was seven. Stated differently, 42 sessions delivering 45–60 minutes of in-home PST, provided by staff trained to adhere to a specific intervention protocol, would be required to delay the onset of one episode of major depression. However, PST would halve the number of those who lost a valued activity. Limiting the effort to those with more carefully defined risk, say only those with insomnia or depressed mood, and refining the intervention to include vision rehabilitation in addition to problem solving might increase effectiveness as well as efficiency (Rovner & Casten, 2008). Nonetheless, this study demonstrates the feasibility and acceptability of such an intervention and the functional outcomes necessary to assess the value (cost saving, burden sparing) of a larger-scale application.

Robinson et al. (2008) also used PST to prevent depression in persons who had experienced a stroke within 90 days of study entry. Consenting stroke patients free of depression were randomly allocated to placebo, escitalopram, or PST. Patients and research staff were blind to medication or placebo status but fully aware of allocation to PST, which was delivered over six sessions within the first 12 weeks. However, unlike those with macular degeneration, the poststroke patients received six "booster" sessions at monthly intervals until the end of the 12 months of observation. Escitalopram was initiated at 5 mg and increased to 10 mg for participants ages 65 and over. At the study's end all three groups improved equally on measures of physical and social function with no change in cognitive performance compared to baseline. Neither were there any differences in adverse reactions between escitalopram, placebo, and PST. Of the 25 cases of depression that emerged, 19 were major, 6 were minor. Of the placebo group, 22.4% became depressed compared to 11.9% of the PST and 8.5% of the escitalopram groups. The placebo group developed major or minor depression 4.5 times more frequently than the escitalopram group and 2.2 times more than those who received PST. Persons with a prior history of a mood disorder were 5.2 times more likely to become depressed. Based only on the frequency of depression onset within the 12 months of observation, 7.2 stroke patients would need to receive escitalopram for 1 year to prevent one episode of depression; 9.1 would need to receive PST. Although one-quarter of the 200 volunteer patients who gave their signed consent to participate dropped out—24 before assessment, 27 before intervention—only 15 (10%) dropped out after entering treatment. Escitalopram and PST were also substantially better than placebo at preventing the onset of generalized anxiety disorder (Mikami et al., 2014).

In summary, low-dose escitalopram provided to persons free of depressive symptoms and anxiety within 90 days after an embolic stroke halved the incidence of depression, substantially reduced the emergence of an anxiety disorder, and was well tolerated by 90% of patients who started the treatment. Although screening for a past history of mood disorders might have selected an added risk indicator, the authors note that prevention for all stroke patients skirts the problem of variable follow-through after screening. Hence it may be easier to treat everyone at risk, provided the intervention is safe and effective, than to spend resources on pursuing individuals at marginally increased risk.

These examples demonstrate an added critical element in prevention. Once a randomized controlled trial proves the efficacy of the intervention, it is then necessary to demonstrate broader applicability across diverse health systems where limited resources, organizational constraints, and patient preferences may present obstacles. Adding an antidepressant regimen to the chemotherapy protocol of all melanoma patients scheduled to receive interferon seems straightforward and inexpensive if a generic antidepressant is prescribed. Identifying socially withdrawn bereaved individuals willing to receive social rhythm therapy is a different matter. To illustrate the point further, consider prophylactic antidepressant therapy immediately after delivery to nondepressed women with a single prior episode of postpartum depression. The antidepressant will significantly reduce the likelihood of a second postpartum episode. However, the probability of remaining depression free following the second delivery is three in four without the antidepressant.

Some new mothers, particularly those who are nursing, may opt to take their chances with recurrence rather than receive medication (Wisner et al., 2004). Characterization of risk indicators, even when they are causal, is only the initial step in establishing when and where preventive efforts should start.

PREVENTION: WHEN AND WITH WHOM?

Studies suggest that the detection of a depressive prodrome—initial symptoms that reliably progress to illness—answers the question of when to begin preventive interventions. Smit et al. (2006) followed a population-based cohort of more than 2,000 adults ages 55 to 85 years for over 3 years to detect the emergence of clinically significant symptoms of depression. Also collected was an array of demographic, functional, biomedical, and psychosocial characteristics thought to predict the incidence of depression among older community residents. This data set allowed them to construct a parsimonious predictive model of risk indicators including female gender, low education, two or more chronic conditions, functional limitations, small social network, and depressive symptoms at baseline. The model accounted for 80% of the risk for clinically significant depression. Depressive symptoms at baseline accounted for half the risk. In order to prevent depressive symptoms from progressing into one clinically significant case, 16 people needed to be treated. However, when the group with baseline depressive symptoms was restricted to include only those with small social networks and functional limitations, the number needed to treat dropped to 5. Reynolds (2008) suggests that a number needed to treat of 3 is the theoretical threshold at which prevention becomes both efficient and compelling. In contrast, Shepherd et al. (1995) estimated that 40 males with hypercholesterolemia would need to be treated for 5 years to prevent one myocardial infarction.

Schoevers et al. (2006) used the same population as Smit et al. but restricted their analyses to persons ages 64–84. They also imposed a categorical (present/absent) diagnostic measure in place of Smit et al.'s (2006) more dimensional (less/more) metric. They then grouped respondents into not depressed, subsyndromally depressed, and major depressive disorder. This provided an opportunity to explore two models of risk for the incidence of major depression. The *selective* prevention model targeted individuals at elevated risk for major depression but with little if any depressive symptomatology at baseline. The *indicated* model targeted those with subsyndromal depression symptoms. In the selective model (those without baseline depressive symptoms), spousal death and chronic illness substantially elevated the risk for developing depression. Within the more restricted indicated model, subsyndromal depression accounted for 40% of the risk. The number of people who needed to be treated to prevent one case of major depression based on the single subsyndromal depression risk factor was 5.8 and accounted for 24% of the new cases. Adding other characteristics elevated the risk to 49%, resulting in an even lower number needed to treat.

The investigators concluded that older persons with symptoms not yet meeting diagnostic criteria may be a segment of the population with a depressive prodrome. Moreover, subsyndromal symptoms may reflect vulnerability to relapse or recurrence among those with a prior unrecognized or unacknowledged depressive episode. Whether subsyndromal depression ignites or reignites a depression syndrome, its choice as a single baseline risk factor minimizes wasted effort directed at persons who may develop symptoms that are likely to remit spontaneously. Indeed the most compelling case for the preventive approach to depression is prevention of recurrence (Reynolds et al., 2006; see also the discussion of family-focused therapy [FFT] in Chapter 4 for a review of interventions to prevent recurrence of bipolar disorder).

Nonetheless, the characterization of multiple risk indicators reduces the number needed to treat. Mast et al. (2004) examined risk indicators associated with cerebrovascular disease including diabetes, hypertension, and heart disease, and their relationship to depression and executive cognitive dysfunction. Older patients were initially assessed at the time of admission to a rehabilitation hospital and 18 months thereafter. Persons with below-average executive function at baseline were more likely to develop depressive symptoms as they accumulated cerebrovascular risk factors. Among those with average or above executive function, the addition of risk factors did not lead to greater levels of depression. Thus the causal risk factor was executive dysfunction with diabetes; hypertension and heart disease were variable markers. However, the exposure rate of older primary care patients to diabetes, hypertension, and heart disease is substantial and may be conceived as a hierarchy of increasing risk for cerebrovascular disease and associated executive dysfunction. In summary, prevention should begin when there are depressive symptoms among populations with cognitive or physical disability and vascular diseases, as described below in the section on collaborative care.

INTERVENTION FOR THE DEPRESSIVE PRODROME: WHERE TO BEGIN?

Although the identification of risk has advanced, prevention in practice remains a problem. In randomized controlled trials of interventions for minor depression or dysthymia, neither PST nor paroxetine was superior to placebo for symptom remission among patients treated in primary care settings (Oxman et al., 2001; Frank et al., 2002).

Allart-van Dam et al. (2007) used an educational approach, the "Coping with Depression" course, for primary care patients with subclinical depressive symptoms. They found no difference in the emergence of major depressive disorder between the intervention and control groups. However, intervention group patients with a lower initial level of depressive symptoms benefited more than controls. Definitions of subclinical, subsyndromal, and minor depression among primary care patients overlap and can be confusing (Lyness et al., 2007), but taken together they are associated with greater costs and as much as a fivefold risk for the subsequent development of a major depressive episode, compared to asymptomatic patients (Pickett et al., 2014a). However, a substantial number—perhaps a majority—of patients in each category will experience a remission of symptoms without intervention. This highlights the need to identify associated primary care patient characteristics that predict a trajectory similar to the models of depression risk developed for older community residents (Smit et al., 2006; Schoevers et al., 2006).

An array of acute medical events or conditions including macular degeneration, stroke (Whyte & Rovner, 2006; Robinson et al., 2008), and myocardial infarction (van't Veer-Tazelaar et al., 2006; Glassman et al., 2002) are markers that have proven to be reliable indicators of depression risk. Self-assessed health and perceived lack of social support may be the simplest and most reliable self-report measures to predict the less benign course (Lyness et al., 2006). An alternative to developing a more reliable prevention model is a stepped-care approach that entails watchful waiting to determine whether initial symptoms persist, followed by education, then PST, then medication (van't Veer-Tazelaar et al., 2006). Mojtabai (2014) argues that the majority older adults in primary care who receive an antidepressant do not meet criteria for the category of depression in which antidepressants are moderately effective. He cites the stepped-care model from the National Institute for Health and Clinical Excellence (2009) *Guidelines for Treatment and*

Management of Depression in Adults as the preferable approach to primary care patients with symptoms of depression. Similarly, Lamers et al. (2006) provide a brief nonpharmacological intervention to older community residents selected for the presence of type 2 diabetes or COPD and mild to moderate depression. Stepped care (see Table 9.1) seems particularly appropriate for prevention of major depression as well.

The American Heart Association considers depression a risk factor for poor prognosis in acute coronary syndromes (Lichtman et al.,

TABLE 9.1. Stepped-Care Model for Primary Care Patients with Symptoms of Depression

Step	Patient presentation[a]	Practitioner response
1	Suspected symptoms of depression	Assessment (Figure 1.1), watchful waiting, support, education, referral if needed for further assessment or more specific intervention
2	Subsyndromal, recurrent brief depression, short-duration depressive episode, depressive episode with insufficient symptoms, adjustment reaction with depressed mood	Self-help educational materials, problem-solving therapy, and behavioral activation (Tables 4.1 and 5.1) face to face or via the Internet, medication (Table 3.1), referral if needed for further assessment or more intensive intervention
3	Symptoms persist despite interventions or meet criteria for major depressive disorder	Medication (Table 3.1), switch or augment medication (Figure 3.1), more intensive psychotherapy, combined medication and psychotherapy, collaborative care (Table 9.2) for depression complicated by comorbid physical illness, referral if needed for further assessment or more intensive intervention
4	Depression complicated by psychosis, bipolar disorder, suicidality, self-neglect	Medication regimen (antidepressant + antipsychotic) specifically for depression with psychosis (Table 3.1) or for bipolar disorder (Table 3.3, Figure 3.3), combined medication with psychotherapy, electroconvulsive therapy, crisis service (emergency admission, see Table 1.4), hospitalization

Note. Based on Mojtabai (2014) and the National Institute for Health and Clinical Excellence (2009).
[a]Symptom definitions from DSM-IV and DSM-5 are found in Table 1.4.

2014). The elevated incidence and mortality of myocardial infarction associated with depression has caused interest in preventive protocols with these patients. However, randomized interventions employing antidepressants (SADHART study; Glassman et al., 2002) and psychotherapy (ENRICHD study; Taylor et al., 2005) have not consistently demonstrated the hoped-for reduction in mortality and subsequent cardiac events despite reductions in depressive symptoms. In contrast, cardiac patients who received antidepressant medication either from their primary care provider or a psychiatrist, either before or after randomization to psychotherapy in the ENRICHD study, experienced significantly less morbidity and mortality (Taylor et al., 2005). Group therapy has also shown promise of reducing depression and anxiety in patients following heart attack (Turner et al., 2014).

There are several arguments for depression prophylaxis among all post– myocardial infarction patients rather than those with depressive symptoms only. First, both antidepressant and psychological treatments in the SADHART and ENRICHD trials may have been started too late to show robust effects. Second, failure to reduce mortality in the intervention groups may be the result of the frequency with which the routine care group also received antidepressants. Third, nonsedating antidepressants are available that inhibit platelet aggregation, do not promote arrhythmias or lower blood pressure, and are relatively free of dangerous drug interactions. Thus the risk of experiencing harm as a result of a preventive antidepressant would be low. Although a strategy of "antidepressants for most if not all" may be reasonable, advances in risk stratification and outcome measures will be required to prove its value. Rovner and Casten's (2008) finding of lasting reduction in disability among macular degeneration patients is one example of more broadly defined meaningful outcomes. The answer to when to start prevention is with the emergence of subsyndromal depression. The answer to where to begin prevention is in primary care settings.

COLLABORATIVE CARE MANAGEMENT: IMPLICATIONS FOR DEPRESSION PREVENTION

A more aggressive approach to depression has emerged that incorporates principles of chronic disease management similar to those employed to improve care and reduce hospitalizations among persons with diabetes or congestive heart failure. These principles are the same as those in the primary care models discussed in Chapter 8 in the context of suicide prevention. In chronic disease management, nursing personnel collaborate with physicians and patients to improve adherence to evidence-based care guidelines. Specialist consultation from cardiologists or endocrinologists is available, but the majority of clinical interaction occurs between patient and nurse. For depression the collaboration integrates a depression care manager, typically nurses with added psychiatric training, psychiatric social workers, or psychologists. Psychiatric consultation is available, but again the majority of clinical interaction occurs between the patient and the care manager rather than with physicians. Comprehensive geriatric evaluation management clinics also employ interdisciplinary teams, including nurses, social workers, and psychologists, to provide chronic disease management, including depression care. Specific elements of the collaborative care model appear in Table 9.2.

Skultety and Zeiss (2006) found both comprehensive geriatric evaluation and the integrated models, which included mental health providers, more effective than routine care in reducing depression in late life. However, because the integrated models were designed specifically for depression and were more likely to focus interventions on severe depression, the models and their outcomes were difficult to compare. Woltman and associates (2012) reviewed a wide array of collaborative chronic care models for mental health disorders across primary, specialty, and behavioral health care settings. Their meta-analysis of collaborative care trials for depression, bipolar disorder, anxiety, and other mental disorders found superior effects for mental and physical health and social role function as well as for depression, with clinically meaningful effect sizes (Cohen's d values 0.20–.033). More recently, the collaborative care model employed in the IMPACT study of primary care patients ages 60 and over who were free of cardiovascular disease at baseline halved the excess risk of subsequent fatal or nonfatal cardiac events (Stewart, Perkins, & Callahan, 2014).

FINANCING PREVENTION

Present arguments for prevention of depression must proceed from analyses of costs compared to benefits. With a focus on primary practice settings, Gilbody, Bower, and Whitty (2006) compared costs and benefits of randomized studies of depression care. Uniformly superior outcomes emerged from studies of collaborative care and case management. Yet

TABLE 9.2. Components of Collaborative Care for Depression

Core	Goal	Methods
Patient self-management	Patients are fully invested and effective partners in management of their depression.	Care manager assists the patient and family with education, problem solving, behavior change, decision making, and motivational aspects of care (see Chapter 4).
Information system	Relevant clinical information about the individual, group, or population of depressed patients is readily available and effortlessly flows to providers.	Feedback about choice of interventions and their outcomes is made available via case registries, reminder systems, and laboratory data.
Delivery system	Work roles for clinicians and support staff redefined to shift from reactive to preventive or anticipatory care. Workforce deployed to support information flow, timely feedback, and patient self-management.	Care managers, therapists, or educators provide psychosocial interventions, ensure clinical information for individual patients is acquired and shared in a timely manner, assess preventive or anticipatory needs of the clinical population.
Provider decision support	Specialist-level input provided for generalists without always sending the patient for a consultation.	Specialists accessible by care managers as well as generalist physicians via onsite or facilitated (online, cellular) interaction.
Community connection	Mobilize the culture and community beyond the health care organization to support the patient.	Exercise programs, peer support groups, faith-based organizations identified.
Organizational support	Leaders in the organization champion the effort with resources necessary for success and sustainability.	Clinical and nonclinical components adequately staffed by personnel trained and monitored in new roles and routines.

Note. Adapted from Woltman et al. (2012). Copyright 2012 by the American Psychiatric Association. Adapted by permission.

incremental improvements in depression care were associated with increments in cost. A collaborative, interdisciplinary approach to depression was cost-effective (valuable) but did not reduce the total costs of care. However, the costs to employers from lessened productivity of depressed employees and their burdened family members were not generally measured.

Concerns over the economic impact of parent care on younger workers have become an added incentive for the prevention of depression in late life (MetLife, 2006). The President's New Freedom Commission on Mental Health (2003) and the National Business Group on Health (Finch, Campbell, & Hardin, 2006) recommended that public and private payers reimburse the collaborative, interdisciplinary model of depression care. Although "care coordination" is reimbursed by Medicare, ongoing telephone consultation and supervision by psychiatrists for depression care managers as practiced in collaborative care models is not. Nonetheless, there are mechanisms through which the approach may be financed (Bachman, Pincus, & Houtsinger, 2006).

Because depressive disorders often go unrecognized in primary care, a considerable reservoir of income may exist to provide for screening and treatment, but also for carefully constructed, modest depression prevention efforts. Although the annual amount may seem excessive, Katon and colleagues (2003) found the excess primary care costs due to major or minor depression were more than $2,000 annually. And Gallo et al. (2005) found that among primary care patients depression is as predictive of mortality as diabetes or coronary heart disease. If depression contributes excess risk of hospitalization, and prevention of depression reduces admissions and attendant costs, the savings might well finance the preventive protocols. Obviously, the savings incentive would apply only to capitated plans and Accountable Care Organizations that have assumed the total costs of care and not to fee-for-service delivery models.

CONCLUSION

Prevention strategies must be added to treatment protocols if the burden of depressive illness is to be substantially reduced. Disabling somatic conditions, most notably stroke, heart attack, and loss of sight, are associated with a predictable prevalence of depressive symptoms and major depressive disorder. Bereavement, executive dysfunction, and trauma also place the older person at increased risk for major depression. Thus in populations selected for screening because of events that place them at elevated risk, and particularly among those with subsyndromal depression, prophylactic antidepressants or psychotherapy may be genuinely preventive. Screening and collaborative protocols to reduce the prevalence and costs of major depressive disorders may generate the income to finance preventive efforts to reduce the incidence as well. If either approach results in a reduced rate of hospitalization due to illnesses that so frequently increase the risk of depression, the coupling of treatment and prevention might prove essential to the financial viability of the care system. For the prevention of depression to become a reality, it must satisfy both individual and collective values. This means preservation of the patient's independence, reduction of the burdens placed on family (and employers), and reduced total costs of care. By placing payments for behavioral health care on par with somatic care, the Mental Health Parity and Addiction Equity Act (2008) promises the necessary element, which, as Patel and Shekhar (2014) argue, is universal mental health care.

Epilogue

As estimated by the Swiss demographer Arthur Imhof and quoted by Martenson (2008), in the year 1600 a resident of Berlin who lived to age 80 could reasonably expect to survive 6 more years on average. In 1980, an 80-year-old Berliner could expect 8 more years of survival. Thus, longevity once one attains advanced age has changed little despite major advances in education, health care, and economic security for older adults. What has changed is the number of persons reaching advanced age, and more importantly, the percentage living independently. More individuals are living to their maximum lifespans more actively than ever.

True enough, the number of dependent elders will increase, but their numbers will be overshadowed by a greater percentage of seniors making an active contribution to the social economy. For example, baby boomers reaching retirement age are staying in the workforce at rates higher than any other recent generation. More than three-quarters of older Americans assess their health as good to excellent. Of Medicare enrollees, 41% report at least one limitation with either instrumental or other activities of daily living. However, only 4% of the older adult population reside in long-term care facilities. Fewer than 20% of older men, but more than 40% of older women live alone (Federal Interagency Forum on Aging-Related Statistics, 2012). Arguments that the needs of older Americans will exceed resources often fail to factor in the contributions older Americans make. Seniors are an asset, not a liability. If we cannot care for seniors today, how will we care for ourselves tomorrow?

PUBLIC POLICY AND AN AGING SOCIETY

While there is cause for hope, current policy and practice regarding depression are misaligned with needs and priorities. In low- to-middle- and higher-income countries, major depressive disorders lead the list of disabling conditions. As measured in YLD, depression outranked alcohol abuse, Alzheimer's disease, COPD, and diabetes, accounting for 14.6% of the total (World Health Organization, 2008). By age 60 cerebrovascular disease, COPD, and dementia rank above depression, but avoidable disability due to depression in each of these disorders is substantial.

As a result, preventing the development and progression of depression-related disability is a public health priority. Yet expenditures for treatment of mental disorders account for 3% of annual Medicare expenses, and half of that is for in-patient care. (Owen, 2007). The mismatch between needs and resources is not associated solely with economic development. As national incomes rise, so do mental health expenditures, but to a plateau far below documented needs (Saxena et al., 2007). This disparity is often explained as evidence of the stigma of mental illness, the belief that mental illness is the result of moral weakness or character flaws, and is neither truly disabling nor treatable.

Prejudicial attitudes toward the aging process in general and older adults in particular further complicate the matter. Otherwise healthy older adults respond as well to antidepressants and to psychotherapy for depression as younger persons (Blazer, 2003). And antidepressant prescription rates have increased substantially for both young and old. Nonetheless, more treatment has not meant better treatment. Here the problem lies not so much with prejudicial attitudes about older adults or mentally ill persons. Rather, in their zeal to emphasize how treatable depression is, mental health advocates (including myself) have neglected to point out how difficult it can be to treat. Equally distressing is the declining number of mental health specialists entering the field of geriatrics (Bragg et al., 2012). Given the lack of available resources for so widespread a disabling condition, it should be no surprise that depression late in life can be difficult to treat.

COLLABORATIVE CARE

As described earlier in this book, recognition of the difficulty inherent in depression treatment has led to a cluster of interventions most commonly called collaborative care (Woltman et al., 2012). Its core element, the depression care manager, was proposed more than a century ago. "If early in the cases of beginning mania and melancholia patients could be placed under the firm, careful management of nurses trained properly to care for them, there would often not be serious outbreaks of mental disturbance that eventually develop under present conditions" ("Mental Disorders and General Practice," 1906/2006). More elements of collaborative care have been elaborated within the last two decades (see Chapter 9 and Table 9.2). The collaborative care concept for mental health disorders is adapted from treatment programs originally developed for diabetes and congestive heart failure, in which patient behavior and provider support are considered as important as symptom assessment and medication management. Although there are established physiological parameters for gauging the adequacy of interventions in diabetes and heart failure, the social psychology of treatment is seen as important as the biology. As a result, in a collaborative care model, a triad or foursome of individuals joins in a collaborative effort to monitor the illness and keep the patient asymptomatic. Typically the patient and primary care provider are joined by a depression care manager, usually a nurse or social worker, with or without involvement of a family member, depending on the model. In addition to the care manager, the model incorporates self-management techniques for the patients, decision support for the primary provider, and an information system that ensures that relevant clinical information is easily accessible.

The care manager assumes much of the responsibility for communication, providing patients with information regarding their illness, self-management techniques, and community resources, as well as being readily available for questions about medications, side effects, and obstacles to recovery. Care managers may also provide a range of psychotherapies and other psychosocial interventions (see Chapters 4 and 5 on psychotherapies and other interventions) depending on the program. Ongoing outcome assessments occur at prearranged intervals. The care manager will also communicate with the primary clinician when obstacles arise, when outcomes are less than desired, or when specialist consultation is indicated. Specialists are available for direct patient consultation when suicidality, psychosis, mania, or treatment resistance complicate the picture; they are also accessible to the care manager and primary care provider on an as-needed basis by phone or online. These indirect consultations can be more numerous and more frequent than face-to-face patient encounters.

Obviously this intensity of communication requires a system in which information flows seamlessly between all parties and there is the logistical support for it to do so. Clinical guidelines, community resources, self-management materials, outcome assessments, appointments, and consultations all need to be available, maintained, and monitored. The electronic medical record is only one element in the system, which requires an array of automation, networking, and communication devices. Collaborative care cannot be sustained without literally reengineering the health care workplace. Furthermore, it takes organizational leadership to invest the time and resources to support new roles and routines with personnel, technology, teaching, and monitoring. However, pilot programs set in motion by the Patient Protection and Affordable Care Act are currently under way to test just such a reengineering of health care delivery and financing. They are called Accountable Care Organizations (ACOs).

Accountable Care Organizations

The Accountable Care Organization (ACO) model provides organizational and funding incentives leading to reorganization of services. Instead of the usual fee-for-service arrangement, Medicare pays the ACO an illness-adjusted set amount for care of a defined population of Medicare beneficiaries. This shifts the ACO's financial incentive from maximizing remunerative services to minimizing costs. Because hospitalization for complications of common chronic conditions such as diabetes, hyperlipidemia, hypertension, and heart failure is institutionally expensive and personally undesirable, there is a shared incentive for patient and ACO alike to avoid hospitalization. Depression interferes with health-related behaviors, complicating self-management of chronic conditions, so it is no surprise that interventions to reduce depression, when combined with care management, lead to superior health outcomes (Katon et al., 2010). What may be surprising is that superior outcomes in quality of life, social role function, and depression are not more expensive in collaborative care than total costs of care in comparison groups (Woltman et al., 2012).

The ACO at Montefiore Medical Center in New York uses all the components of collaborative care, including an electronic health record accessible across acute-care and ambulatory sites and standardized treatment guidelines that prompt providers to "treat to target"—meaning to aim their interventions to accomplish quantifiable outcomes. The targets include specified ranges for blood pressure, blood glucose (hemo-globin A1c), low-density lipoprotein (LDL cholesterol), and depressive symptoms. Using these ranges, clinicians determine whether they need to initiate, intensify, or moderate treatment. The ranges thus support the decision-making process with unequivocal guidance to the patient and provider. The Montefiore ACO uses both medical and behavioral health care managers; these nurses and social workers already have the requisite skills and orientation. However, the ACO redeploys them as a collaborative "synergy" team. Much of the contact between patients and managers, including psychotherapy, is accomplished by phone. Consultation with cardiologists, diabetologists, and psychiatrists may be triggered when targets are not met through behavioral activation (see Chapter 4 on psychotherapy) or adjustment of medications.

The potential benefits of the ACO approach go beyond management of existing illnesses. Age-related functional changes including frailty, accelerated loss of bone and muscle mass, apathy, lack of socialization, and cognitive decline represent potentially modifiable transitions to disease states. Interventions developed from animal models that alter each of these transitional states promise to extend the active lifespan, such that dependency due to illness in old age could be reduced to a minimum (Hamerman, 2010). Similarly, in the treatment of depression, identifying ways to promote functional integrity is one of the most important means of increasing the chances of sustained recovery. This is particularly important because depressed older persons are less likely than younger persons to recognize depression symptoms as an illness (Alexopoulos et al., 2004). They are also less likely to present depression as an initial complaint to their primary care physicians despite the fact primary care providers treat the majority of depressed persons.

CONCLUSION

The complexity of depressive syndromes across the adult lifespan should not cause alarm. Rather, it promises multiple avenues of engagement, with scientific evidence to support the choice of interventions, health policy to provide incentives, and examples of leadership to implement the necessary platform. The extent to which public demand will translate the science of depression care into services in the future remains to be seen. But that is no reason for professional passivity. Make use of the information in this book, so you can deliver better care now.

References

Abbott RD, White LR, Ross GW, et al. (2004). Walking and dementia in physically capable elderly men. *JAMA, 292,* 1447–1461.

Agronin ME. (2009, January/February). Psychotherapy for older patients: An interview with AAGP member Patrician Areán, PhD. *Geriatric Psychiatry News, 5.*

Aizenstein HJ, Andreescu C, Edelman KL, et al. (2011). FMRI correlates of white matter hyperintensities in late-life depression. *Am J Psychiatry, 168*(10), 1075–1082.

Alexopoulos GS, Katz IR, Bruce ML, et al. (2005a). Remission in depressed geriatric primary care patients: A report from the Prospect Study. *Am J Psychiatry, 162,* 718–724.

Alexopoulos GS, Kiosses DN, Choi SJ, et al. (2002). Frontal white matter microstructure and treatment response of late-life depression: A preliminary study. *Am J Psychiatry, 159*(11), 1929–1932.

Alexopoulos GS, Kiosses DN, Heo M, et al. (2005b). Executive dysfunction and the course of geriatric depression. *Biol Psychiatry, 58*(3), 204–210.

Alexopoulos GS, Kiosses DN, Murphy C, et al. (2004). Executive dysfunction, heart disease burden, and remission of geriatric depression. *Neuropsychopharmacology, 29*(12), 2278–2284.

Alexopoulos GS, Meyers BS, Young RC, et al. (1997). Clinically defined vascular depression. *Am J Psychiatry, 154*(4), 562–565.

Alexopoulos GS, Meyers BS, Young RC, et al. (2000). Executive dysfunction and long-term outcomes of geriatric depression. *Arch Gen Psychiatry, 57*(3), 285–290.

Alexopoulos GS, Morimoto SS. (2011). The inflammation hypothesis in geriatric depression. *Int J Geriatr Psychiatry, 26,* 1109–1118.

Alexopoulos GS, Murphy CF, Gunning-Dixon FM, et al. (2008). Microstructural white matter abnormalities and remission of geriatric depression. *Am J Psychiatry, 165*(2), 238–244.

Alexopoulos GS, Raue P, Areán PA. (2003). Problem solving therapy versus supportive therapy in geriatric major depression with executive dysfunction. *Am J Geriatr Psychiatry, 11*, 46–52.

Alexopoulos GS, Reynolds CF III, Bruce M, et al. (2009). Reducing suicidal ideation and depression in older primary care patients: 24-month outcomes of the PROSPECT study. *Am J Psychiatry, 166*, 882–890.

Allart-van Dam E, Hosman CM, Hoogduin CA, et al. (2007). Prevention of depression in subclinically depressed adults: Follow-up effects on the "Coping with Depression" course. *J Affect Disord, 97*(1–3), 219–228.

Allen K, Cull A, Sharpe M. (2003). Diagnosing major depression in medical outpatients: Acceptability of telephone interviews. *J Psychosom Res, 55*, 385–387.

Altman J, Das GD. (1965). Autoradiographic and histological evidence of postnatal hippocampal neurogenesis in rats. *J Comp Neurol, 124*, 319–335.

American Medical Association. (2008). *Physician resource guide to patient self-management support*. Chicago: Author.

American Psychiatric Association. (1994). *Diagnostic and statistical manual of mental disorders* (4th ed.). Washington, DC: Author.

American Psychiatric Association. (2000). *Diagnostic and statistical manual of mental disorders* (4th ed., text rev.). Washington, DC: Author.

American Psychiatric Association. (2000). Practice guideline for treatment of patients with major depressive disorder (revision). *Am J Psychiatry, 157*(Suppl. 4), 1–45.

American Psychiatric Association. (2013). *Diagnostic and statistical manual of mental disorders* (5th ed.). Arlington, VA: Author.

Andersen J, Aabro E, Gulmann N, et al. (1980). Anti-depressive treatment in Parkinson's disease: A controlled trial of the effect of nortriptyline in patients with Parkinson's disease treated with l-dopa. *Acta Neurol Scand, 62*, 210–219.

Anderson BJ, Rapp DN, Back DH, et al. (2000). Exercise influences spatial learning in the radial arm maze. *Physiol Behav, 70*, 425–429.

Andreescu C, Lenze EJ, Dew MA, et al. (2007). Effect of comorbid anxiety on treatment response and relapse risk in late-life depression: Controlled study. *Br J Psychiatry, 190*, 344–349.

Andreescu C, Mulsant BH, Houck PR, et al. (2008). Empirically derived decision trees for the treatment of late-life depression. *Am J Psychiatry, 165*(7), 855–862.

Andreescu C, Mulsant BH, Peasley-Miklus C. (2007). Persisting low use of antipsychotics in the treatment of major depressive disorder with psychotic features. *J Clin Psychiatry, 68*(2), 194–200.

Aneshensel CS, Freriches RR, Clark VA, et al. (1982). Measuring depression in the community: A comparison of telephone and personal interviews. *Public Opinion Quarterly, 46*, 110–121.

Angst J, Presig M. (1995). Outcome of a clinical cohort of unipolar, bipolar, and schizoaffective patients: Results of a prospective study from 1959 to 1985. *Schweiz Arch Neurol Psychiatry, 146,* 17–23.

Areán PA. (2004). Psychosocial treatments for depression in the elderly. *Primary Psychiatry, 11,* 48–53.

Areán PA, Ayalon L, Chengshi J, et al. (2008b). Integrated specialty mental health care among older minorities improves access but not outcomes: Results of the PRISMe study. *Int J Geriatr Psychiatry, 23,* 1086–1092.

Areán PA, Cook BL. (2002). Psychotherapy and combined psychotherapy/pharmacotherapy for late life depression. *Biol Psychiatry, 52,* 293–303.

Areán PA, Hegel M, Vannoy S, et al. (2008a). Effectiveness of problem-solving therapy for older, primary care patients with depression: Results from the IMPACT project. *Gerontologist, 48*(3), 311–323.

Areán PA, Raue P, Mackin RS, et al. (2010). Problem-solving therapy and supportive therapy in older adults with major depression and executive dysfunction. *Am J Psychiatry, 167*(11), 1391–1398.

Aschbacher K, Epel E, Wolkowitz OM, et al. (2012). Maintenance of a positive outlook during acute stress protects against pro-inflammatory reactivity and future depressive symptoms. *Brain Behav Immun, 26*(2), 346–352.

Bachman J, Pincus HA, Houtsinger JK, et al. (2006). Funding mechanisms for depression care management: Opportunities and challenges. *Gen Hosp Psychiatry, 28,* 278–288.

Baltes PB, Baltes MM. (1990). Psychological perspective on successful aging: The model of selective optimization with compensation. In PB Baltes & MM Baltes (Eds.), *Successful aging: Perspective from the behavioral sciences* (pp. 1–34). New York: Cambridge University Press.

Bandura A. (1986). *Social foundations of thought and action: A social cognitive theory.* Englewood Cliffs, NJ: Prentice Hall.

Barbui C, Campomori A, D'Avanzo B, et al. (1999). Antidepressant drug use in Italy since the introduction of selective serotonin reuptake inhibitors (SSRIs): National trends, regional differences and impact on suicide rates. *Soc Psychiatry Psychiatr Epidemiol, 34,* 152–156.

Barlow DA, Craske MG. (1989). *Mastery of your anxiety and panic.* Albany, NY: Graywind.

Bartle SH, Aldin P, Green MR, et al. (1995). Attitudes of physicians towards psychiatry: Some criticism which psychiatrists might modify. *Berkshire Medical Journal, 3,* 7–10.

Batterham PJ, Christensen H. (2012). Longitudinal risk profiling for suicidal thoughts and behaviors in a community cohort using decision trees. *J Affect Disord, 142,* 306–314.

Beach SRH, Fincham FD, Katz J. (1996). Social support in marriage: A cognitive perspective. In GR Pierce, BR Sarason, IG Sarason (Eds.), *Handbook of social support and the family* (pp. 43–64). New York: Plenum Press.

Beard JR, Cerdá M, Blaney S, et al. (2009). Neighborhood characteristics and change in depressive symptoms among older residents of New York City. *Am J Public Health, 99*(7), 1308–1314.

Beautrais AL. (2002). A case control study of suicide and attempted suicide in older adults. *Suicide Life Threat Behav, 32,* 1–9.

Beck AT. (1976). *Cognitive therapy and the emotional disorders.* New York: International Universities Press.

Beck AT, Kovacs M, Weissman A. (1979). Assessment of suicidal intention: The scale for suicidal ideation. *J Consult Clin Psychol, 47,* 343–352.

Beekman ATF, Geerlings SW, Deeg D, et al. (2002). The natural history of late-life depression: A 6 year prospective study in the community. *Arch Gen Psychiatry, 59,* 605–611.

Begle AM, Strachan M, Cisler JM, et al. (2011). Elder mistreatment and emotional symptoms among older adults in a largely rural population: The South Carolina elder mistreatment study. *J Interpers Violence, 26*(11), 2321–2332.

Benton AL, Hamsher K de S, Sivan AB. (1994). Controlled Oral Word Association Test (COWAT). In *Multilingual aphasia examination* (3rd ed.). Iowa City, IA: AJA Associates.

Berger AK, Fratiglioni L, Forsell Y, et al. (1999). The occurrence of depressive symptoms in the preclinical phase of AD: A population-based study. *Neurology, 53,* 1998–2002.

Berkman LF, Blumenthal J, Burg M, et al. (2003). Effects of treating depression and low perceived social support on clinical events after myocardial infarction: The Enhancing Recovery in Coronary Heart Disease Patients (ENRICHD) Randomized Trial. *JAMA, 289,* 3106–3116.

Betan E, Heim AK, Zittel Conklin C, et al. (2005). Countertransference phenomena and personality pathology in clinical practice: An empirical investigation. *Am J Psychiatry, 162,* 833–835.

Bischoff-Ferrari H. (2009). Vitamin D: What is an adequate vitamin D level and how much supplementation is necessary? *Best Pract Res Clin Rheumatol, 23*(6), 789–795.

Bjelakovic G, Nikolova D, Gluud LL, et al. (2008). Antioxidant supplements for prevention of mortality in healthy participants and patients with various diseases. *Cochrane Database Syst Rev, 2,* CD007176.

Blazer DG. (2003). Depression in late life: Review and commentary. *J Gerontol A Biol Sci Med Sci, 58,* 249–265.

Blazer DG, Wu L-T. (2009). The epidemiology of at-risk and binge drinking among middle-aged and elderly community adults: National Survey on Drug Use and Health. *Am J Psychiatry, 166,* 1162–1169.

Bogner HR, Morales HK, Reynolds CE, et al. (2012). Course of depression and mortality among older primary care patients. *Am J Geriatr Psychiatry, 20,* 895–903.

Bohlmeijer E, Roemer M, Cuijpers P, et al. (2007). The effects of reminiscence on psychological well-being in older adults: A meta-analysis. *Aging Ment Health, 11,* 291–300.

Bolger N, Zuckerman A, Kessler RC. (2000). Invisible support and adjustment to stress. *J Pers Soc Psychol, 79,* 953–961.

Bolland MJ, Avenell A, Baron JA, et al. (2010). Effect of calcium supplements on risk of myocardial infarction and cardiovascular events: Meta-analysis. *BMJ, 341,* 3691–3699.

Bonanno GA, Galea S, Bucciarelli A, et al. (2006). Psychological resilience after disaster: New York City in the aftermath of the September 11th terrorist attack. *Psychol Sci, 17*, 181–186.

Boss P, Caron W, Horbal J, et al. (1990). Predictors of depression in caregivers of dementia patients: Boundary ambiguity and mastery. *Family Process, 29*, 245–254.

Bosworth HB, McQuoid MS, George LK, et al. (2002). Time-to-remission from geriatric depression: Psychosocial and clinical factors. *Am J Geriatr Psychiatry, 10*, 551–559.

Bowden CL, Asnis GM, Bently LD, et al. (2004). Safety and tolerability of lamotrigine for bipolar. *Drug Saf, 27*(3), 173–184.

Boyette LW, Sharon BF, Brandon J. (1997). A follow-up study on the effect of strength training in aging. *J Nutr Health Aging, 1*, 109–1113.

Bragg EJ, Warshaw GA, Cheong J, et al. (2012). National survey of geriatric psychiatry fellowship programs: Comparing findings in 2006/07 and 2001/02 from the American Geriatrics Society and Association of Directors of Geriatric Academic Programs' Geriatrics Workforce Policy Studies Center. *J Am Geriatr Soc, 60*(8), 1540–1545.

Brandon J, Sharon BF, Boyette LW. (1997). Effects of a training program on blood pressure in aging. *J Nutr Health Aging, 1*, 98–102.

Bray GA. (1999). Nutrition and obesity: Prevention and treatment. *Nutr Metab Cardiovasc Dis, 9*(Suppl. 4), 21–32.

Brent DA, Oquendo MA, Birmaher B, et al. (2002). Familial pathways to early-onset suicide attempts: Risk for suicidal behavior in offspring of mood-disordered suicide attempters. *Arch Gen Psychiatry, 59*(9), 1037–1044.

Brown GK, Ten Have TR, Henriques GR, et al. (2005). Cognitive therapy for the prevention of suicide attempts: A randomized controlled trial. *JAMA, 294*, 563–570.

Bruce ML, Ten Have TR, Reynolds CF III, et al. (2004). Reducing suicidal ideation and depressive symptoms in depressed older primary care patients: A randomized controlled trial. *JAMA, 291*, 1081–1091.

Buchanan D, Tourigny-Rivard MF, Cappeliez P, et al. (2006). National guidelines for seniors' mental health: The assessment of and treatment of depression. *Can J Psychiatry, 9*(Suppl. 2), S52–S58

Büchtemann D, Luppa M, Bramesfeld A, et al. (2012). Incidence of late-life depression: A systematic review. *J Affect Disord, 142*(1–3), 172–179.

Buhr G, Bales CW. (2009). Nutritional supplements for older adults: Review and recommendations—Part I. *J Nutr Elder, 28*(1), 5–29.

Buhr G, Bales CW. (2010). Nutritional supplements for older adults: Review and recommendations—Part II. *J Nutr Elder, 29*(1), 42–71.

Burns DD. (1989). *The feeling good handbook: Using the new mood therapy in everyday life.* New York: Morrow.

Butler RN. (1963). The life review: An intervention of reminiscence in the aged. *Psychiatry, 26*, 65–70.

Butler RN.(1996). Lost in the campaign rhetoric. Today's decisions on Social Security and Medicare will steer 'the era of longevity'. *Geriatrics, 51*(11), 9–10.

Butler RN, Lewis MI. (1977). *Aging and mental health: Positive psychosocial approaches*. St. Lewis, MO: CV Mosby.

Byers AL, Yaffe K, Covinsky KE, et al. (2010). High occurrence of mood and anxiety disorders among older adults: The National Comorbidity Survey Replication. *Arch Gen Psychiatry, 67*(5), 489–496.

Caine ED. (2012). Suicide prevention is a winnable battle. *Am J Public Health, 102*(Suppl. 1), S4–S5.

Calabrese JR, Bowden CL, Sachs GS, et al. (1999). A double-blind placebo-controlled study of lamotrigine in outpatients with bipolar I depression. *J Clin Psychiatry, 60*, 79–88.

Calfas KJ, Zabinski MF, Rupp J. (2000). Practical nutrition assessment in primary care settings: A review. *Am J Prev Med, 18*(4), 289–299.

Callahan CM, Boustani MA, Unverzagt FW, et al. (2006). Effectiveness of collaborative care for older adults with Alzheimer disease in primary care: A randomized controlled trial. *JAMA, 295*, 2148–2157.

Cameron HA, Gould E. (1994). Adult neurogenesis is regulated by adrenal steroids in the dentate gyrus. *Neuroscience, 61*, 203–209.

Capistrant BD, Berkman LF, Glymour MM. (2013, June 20). Does duration of spousal caregiving affect risk of depression onset? Evidence from the Health and Retirement Study. *Am J Geriatr Psychiatry, 22*(8), 766–770.

Capistrant BD, Moon JR, Berkman LF, et al. (2012). Current and long-term spousal caregiving and onset of cardiovascular disease. *J Epidemiol Community Health, 66*(10), 951–956.

Carlsten A, Waern M, Ekedahl A, et al. (2001). Antidepressant medication and suicide in Sweden. *Pharmacoepidemiol Drug Saf, 10*, 525–530.

Carney RM, Freedland KE. (2009). Treatment-resistant depression and mortality after acute coronary syndrome. *Am J Psychiatry, 166*, 410–417.

Cavanagh JTO, Carson AJ, Sharpe M, et al. (2003). Psychological autopsy studies of suicide: A systematic review. *Psychological Medicine, 33*, 395–405.

Centers for Disease Control and Prevention (2010). Current depression among adults—United States, 2006 and 2008. *MMWR Morb Mortal Wkly Rep, 59*(38), 1229–1235.

Centers for Disease Control and Prevention. (2014). Web-based Injury Statistics Query and Reporting System (WISQARS). Available at *www.cdc.gov/ncipc/wisqars/default.htm*.

Centers for Disease Control and Prevention & Merck Company Foundation. (2007). *The state of aging and health in America*. Whitehouse Station, NJ: Authors.

Chan AS, Ho Y-C, Cheung M-C, et al. (2005). Association between mind-body and cardiovascular exercises and memory in older adults. *J Am Geriatr Soc, 53*, 1754–1760.

Chapman DP, Perry GS. (2008). Depression as a major component of public health for older adults. *Prev Chronic Dis, 5*(1), A22.

Charles ST, Mather M, Carstensen LL. (2003). Aging and emotional Memory: The forgettable nature of negative images for older adults. *J Exp Psychol Gen, 132*(2), 310–324.

Choi J, Lisanby SH, Medalia A, et al. (2011). A conceptual introduction to cognitive remediation for memory deficits associated with right unilateral electroconvulsive therapy. *J ECT, 27*(4), 286–291.

Coates RJ, Bowen DJ, Kristal AR, et al. (1999). The Women's Health Trial Feasibility Study in Minority Populations: Changes in dietary intakes. *Am J Epidemiol, 149*(12), 1104–1112.

Cohen D, Eisdorfer C. (1988) Depression in family members caring for a relative with Alzheimer's disease. *J Am Geriatr Soc, 36*(10), 885–889.

Colcombe SJ, Erickson KI, Scalf PE, et al. (2006). Aerobic exercise increases brain volume in aging humans. *J Gerontol A Biol Sci Med Sci, 61*, 1166–1170.

Colcombe SJ, Kramer AF. (2003). Fitness effects on cognitive function of older adults: A meta-analytic study. *Psychol Sci, 14*, 125–130.

Colemon YR, Kennedy GJ, Mudge R, et al. (2008, March). *Depression treatment of African Americans within a primary care setting.* Poster presentation at the annual meeting of the American Association for Geriatric Psychiatry, Orlando, FL.

Collins PY, Patel V, Joestl SS, et al. (2011). Grand challenges in global mental health. *Nature, 475*, 27–30.

Colman RJ, Anderson RM, Johnson SC, et al. (2009). Caloric restriction delays disease onset and mortality in rhesus monkeys. *Science, 325*, 201–204.

Conwell Y. (2009). Suicide prevention in later life: A glass half full, or half empty. *Am J Psychiatry, 166*(8), 845–848.

Conwell Y, Duberstein PR, Caine ED. (2002). Risk factors for suicide in later life. *Biol Psychiatry, 52*, 193–204.

Conwell Y, Olsen K, Caine ED, et al. (1991). Suicide in later life: Psychological autopsy findings. *Int Psychogeriatr, 3*, 59–66.

Conwell Y, Van Orden K, Caine ED. (2011). Suicide in older adults. *Psychiatr Clin North Am, 34*(2), 451–468.

Cooney GM, Dwan K, Greig CA, et al. (2013). Exercise for depression. *Cochrane Database Syst Rev, 9*, CD004366.

Cooney LM, Kennedy GJ, Hawkins KA, et al. (2004). Who can stay at home: Assessing the capacity to choose to live in the community. *Arch Intern Med, 164*, 357–360.

Coupland C, Dhiman P, Morriss R, et al. (2011). Antidepressant use and risk of adverse outcomes in older people: Population based cohort study. *BMJ, 343*, d4551.

Cuijpers P, van Straten A, Bohlmeijer E, et al. (2010). The effects of psychotherapy for adult depression are overestimated: A meta-analysis of study quality and effect size. *Psychol Med, 40*(2), 211–223.

Cutler DM, Ghosh K, Landrum MB. (2013, July). *Evidence for significant compression of morbidity in the elderly U.S. population* (National Bureau of Economic Research Working Paper 19268). Retrieved August 29, 2013, from *www.nber.org/papers/w19268*.

Darien-Alexis L, Ecclestone NA, Myers AM, et al. (1999). A randomized outcome evaluation of group exercise programs in long-term care institutions. *J Gerontol A Biol Sci Med Sci, 54A*, M621–M628.

Datto CJ, Thompon R, Horowitz D, et al. (2003). The pilot study of a telephone disease management program for depression. *Gen Hosp Psychiatry, 25*, 169–177.

Davis MI. (2008). Ethanol-BDNF interactions: Still more questions than answers. *Pharmacol Ther, 118*, 36–57.

DeBattista C, Lembke A. (2008). Challenges in differentiating and diagnosing psychotic depression: Phenomenology and the pursuit of optimal treatment. *Primary Psychiatry, 25*(4), 59–64.

DeGruy FV. (2006). A note on the partnership between psychiatry and primary care. *Am J Psychiatry, 163*, 1487–1489.

Dew MA, Reynolds CF, Houck PR, et al. (1997). Temporal profiles of the course of depression during treatment: Predictors of pathways toward recovery in the elderly. *Arch Gen Psychiatry, 54*, 1016–1024.

Dew MA, Whyte EM, Lenze EJ, et al. (2007). Recovery from major depression in older adults receiving augmentation of antidepressant pharmacotherapy. *Am J Psychiatry, 164*(6), 892–899.

Dillehay RC, Sandys MR. (1990). Caregivers for Alzheimer's patients: What we are learning from research. *Int J Aging Hum Dev, 30*(4), 263–285.

Dimidjian S, Hollon SD, Dobson KS, et al. (2006). Randomized trial of behavioral activation, cognitive therapy, and antidepressant medication in the acute treatment of adults with major depression. *J Consult Clin Psychol, 74*(4), 658–670.

Dobson KS, Hollon SD, Dimidjian S, et al. (2008). Randomized trial of behavioral activation, cognitive therapy, and antidepressant medication in the prevention of relapse and recurrence in major depression. *J Consult Clin Psychol, 76*(3), 468–477.

Dolder CR, Depp CA, Jeste DV. (2007). Biological treatments of bipolar disorder in later life. In M Sajatovic & FC Blow (Eds.), *Bipolar disorder in later life* (pp. 71–93). Baltimore: Johns Hopkins University Press.

Dolenc TJ, Barnes RD, Hayes DL, et al. (2004). Electroconvulsive therapy in patients with cardiac pacemakers and implantable cardioverter defibrillators. *Pacing Clin Electrophysiol, 27*(9), 1257–1263.

Driscoll HC, Basinski J, Mulsant BH, et al. (2005). Late-onset major depression: Clinical and treatment-response variability. *Int J Geriatr Psychiatry, 20*, 661–667.

Drye LT, Martin BK, Frangakis CE, et al. (2011). Do treatment effects vary among differing baseline depression criteria in Depression in Alzheimer's disease Study–2 (DIADS-2)? *Int J Geriatr Psychiatry, 26*(6), 573–583.

Dukakis K, Tye L. (2006). *Shock: The healing power of electroconvulsive therapy.* New York: Penguin.

Dunn AL, Trivedi MH, O'Neal HA. (2001). Physical activity dose-response effects on outcomes of depression and anxiety. *Med Sci Sports Exerc, 33*, S587–S597.

Eden J, Maslow K, Le M, et al. (2012). *The mental health and substance use workforce for older adults: In whose hands?* Washington, DC: National Academies Press.

Ehlers CL, Frank E, Kupfer DJ. (1988). Social zeitgebers and biological rhythms: A unified approach to understanding the etiology of depression. *Arch Gen Psychiatry, 45,* 948–952.

Engel CC, Oxman T, Yamamoto C, et al. (2008). RESPECT-Mil: Feasibility of a systems-level collaborative care approach to depression and post-traumatic stress disorder in military primary care. *Mil Med, 173,* 935–940.

ENRICHD Investigators. (2001). Enhancing recovery in coronary heart disease patients (ENRICHD): Rationale and design. *Psychosom Med, 63,* 747–755.

Erickson KI, Voss MW, Prakash RS, et al. (2011). Exercise training increases size of hippocampus and improves memory. *Proc Natl Acad Sci USA, 15, 108*(7), 3017–3022.

Fang F, Fall K, Mittleman MA, et al. (2012). Suicide and cardiovascular death after a cancer diagnosis. *N Engl J Med, 366*(14), 1310–1318.

Fava M, Mischoulon D, Rosenbaum J. (1998). Augmentation strategies for failed SSRI treatment: A survey of the Massachusetts General Hospital Clinical Psychopharmacology Unit. *American Society of Clinical Psychopharmacology Progress Notes, 9,* 7.

Fava M, Rush AJ, Trivedi MH, et al. (2003). Background and rationale for the Sequenced Treatment Alternatives to Relieve Depression (STAR*D) study. *Psychiatr Clin N Am, 26,* 457–494.

Fava M, Rush AJ, Wisniewski SR, et al. (2006). A comparison of mirtazapine and nortriptyline following two consecutive failed medication treatments for depressed outpatients: A STAR*D report. *Am J Psychiatry, 163,* 1161–1172.

Federal Interagency Forum on Aging-Related Statistics. (2012). *Older Americans 2012: Key Indicators of Well-Being.* Washington, DC: U.S. Government Printing Office. Available at *www.agingstats.gov.*

Fiatarone MA, O'Neill EF, Ryan ND, et al. (1994). Exercise and nutritional supplementation for physical frailty in very elderly people. *N Engl J Med,* 1769–1775.

Fillit H, Butler, RN. (2009). The frailty identity crisis. *J Am Geriatr Soc, 57,* 348–352.

Finch R, Campbell KP, Harbin H. (2005, December 16). An employer's guide to behavioral health services, National Business Group on Health. Retrieved March 25, 2009, from *www.businessgrouphealth.org/pub/f3139c4c-2354-d714-512d-355c09ddcbc4.*

Fink M. (1984). Meduna and the origins of convulsive therapy. *Am J Psychiatry, 41*(9), 1034–1041.

Finlay IG, George R. (2011). Legal physician-assisted suicide in Oregon and the Netherlands: Evidence concerning the impact on patients in vulnerable groups—another perspective on Oregon's data. *J Med Ethics, 37*(3), 171–174.

Floyd M, Scogin F, McKendree-Smith NL, et al. (2004). Cognitive therapy for depression: A comparison of individual psychotherapy and bibliotherapy for depressed older adults. *Behavior Modification, 28,* 297–318.

Ford AH, Flicker L, McCaul K, et al. (2010). The B-VITAGE trial: A randomized trial of homocysteine lowering treatment of depression in later life. *Trials, 11*, 8.

Frances A. (2012, December 2). DSM5 is guide not bible, ignore its ten worst changes. *Psychology Today* blog. Available at *www.psychologytoday.com/blog/dsm5-in-distress/201212/dsm-5-is-guide-not-bible-ignore-its-ten-worst-changes.*

Frank E, Frank N, Cornes C, et al. (1993). Interpersonal psychotherapy in the treatment of late-life depression. In GI Klerman & MM Weissman (Eds.), *New applications of interpersonal psychotherapy* (pp. 167–198). Washington, DC: American Psychiatric Press.

Frank E, Kupfer DJ, Thase ME, et al. (2005). Two-year outcomes for interpersonal and social rhythm therapy in individuals with bipolar I disorder. *Arch Gen Psychiatry, 62*, 996–1004.

Frank E, Rucci P, Katon W, et al. (2002). Correlates of remission in primary care patients treated for minor depression. *Gen Hosp Psychiatry, 24*, 12–19.

Freeman MP, Fava M, Lake J, et al. (2010). Complementary and alternative medicine in major depressive disorder: The American Psychiatry Association task force report. *J Clin Psychiatry, 71*(6), 669–681.

Fries JF, Bruce B, Chakravarty E. (2011). Compression of morbidity 1980–2011: A focused review of paradigms and progress. *J Aging Res.*

Fritsch T, Smyth KA, McClendon MJ, et al. (2005). Associations between dementia/mild cognitive impairment and cognitive performance and activity levels in youth. *J Am Geriatr Society, 53*, 1111–1532.

Gallagher DE, Thompson LW. (1982). Differential effectiveness of psychotherapies for the treatment of major depressive disorders in older adult patients. *Psychotherapy: Theory, Research, and Practice, 19*, 482–490.

Gallagher-Thompson DE, Coon DW. (2007). Evidence-based treatments for distress in family caregivers of older adults. *Psychol Aging, 22*(1), 37–51.

Gallagher-Thompson D, Steffen AM. (1994). Comparative effects of cognitive-behavioral and brief psychodynamic psychotherapies for depressed family caregivers. *J Consult Clin Psychol, 62*(3), 543–549.

Gallagher-Thompson DE, Thompson LW. (1995). Psychotherapy with older adults in theory and practice. In B. Bonger & L. Beutler (Eds.), *Comprehensive textbook of psychotherapy* (pp. 357–379). New York: Oxford University Press.

Gallo JJ, Bogner HR, Morales KH, et al. (2005). Depression, cardiovascular disease, diabetes and 2-year mortality among older primary care patients. *Amer J Geriatr Psychiatry, 13*, 748–755.

Gardner BK, O'Connor DW. (2008). A review of the cognitive effects of electroconvulsive therapy in older adults. *J ECT, 24*(1), 961–966.

Gaugler JE, Rith DL, Haley WE, et al. (2008). Can counseling and support reduce burden and depressive symptoms in caregivers of people with Alzheimer's disease during the transition to institutionalization? Results from the New York University caregiver intervention study. *J Am Geriatr Society, 56*(3), 421–428.

A generation at risk: Breaking the cycle of senior suicide: Hearings before the Special Committee on Aging, U.S. Senate (2006, September 14) (testimony of Gordon H. Smith, chairman), *http://aging.senate.gov/public/ index.cfm?Fuseaction=Hearings.Detail&HearingID=188.*

A generation at risk: Breaking the cycle of senior suicide: Hearings before the Special Committee on Aging, U.S. Senate (2006, September 14) (testimony of Senator Herb Kohl), *http://aging.senate.gov/hearings/generation- at-risk-breaking-the-cycle-of-senior-suicide.*

George LK. (1994). Caregiver burden and well-being: An elusive distinction. *Gerontologist, 34*(1), 6–7.

Ghisletta P, Bickel J-F, Lövden M. (2006). Does activity engagement protect against cognitive decline in old age? Methodological and analytical considerations. *J Gerontol B Psychol Sci Soc Sci, 61*, P253–P261.

Gilbody S, Bower P, Whitty P. (2006). Costs and consequences of enhanced care for depression: Systematic review of randomized economic evaluations. *Br J Psychiatry, 189*, 297–308.

Gildengers AG, Butters MA, Chisolm D, et al. (2007). Cognitive functioning and instrumental activities of daily living in late-life bipolar disorder. *Am J Geriatr Psychiatry, 15*(2), 174–179.

Gildengers AG, Houck PR, Mulsant BH, et al. (2002). Course and rate of antidepressant response in the very old. *J Affect Disord, 69*, 177–184.

Gildengers AG, Houck PR, Mulsant BH, et al. (2005). Trajectories of treatment response in late-life depression: Psychosocial and clinical correlates. *J Clin Psychopharmacol, 25*(Suppl. 1), S8–S13.

Gläschera J, Adolphsa R, Damasiod H, et al. (2012). Lesion mapping of cognitive control and value-based decision making in the prefrontal cortex. *Proc Natl Acad Sci, 109*(36), 14681–14686.

Glassman AH, O'Connor CM, Califf RM, et al. (2002). Sertraline treatment of major depression in patients with acute MI or unstable angina. *JAMA, 288*, 701–709.

Glick ID. (2004). Adding psychotherapy to pharmacotherapy: Data, benefits, and guidelines for integration. *Am J Psychother, 58*, 186–208.

Goldberg JF, Perlis RH, Ghaemi SN, et al. (2007). Adjunctive antidepressant use and symptomatic recovery among bipolar depressed patients with concomitant manic symptoms: Findings from the STEP-BD. *Am J Psychiatry, 164*(9), 1348–1355.

Goldney RD, Wilson D, Grande ED, et al. (2000). Suicidal ideation in a random community sample: Attributable risk due to depression and psychosocial and traumatic events. *Aust NZ J Psychiat, 43*, 98–106.

Grandin LD, Alloy LB, Abramson LY. (2006). The social zeitgeber theory, circadian rhythms, and mood disorders: Review and evaluation. *Clin Psychol Rev, 26*, 679–694.

Greenberg LS, Rice LN, Elliot R. (1993). *Facilitating emotional change: The moment-by-moment process.* New York: Guilford Press.

Grotjahn M. (1955). Analytic psychotherapy with the elderly. *Psychoanal Rev, 42*, 419–427.

Gum A, Areán PA. (2004). Current status of psychotherapy for mental disorders in the elderly. *Curr Psychiatry Rep, 6*, 32–28.

Haas AP, Hendin GE. (1983). Suicide among older people: Projections for the future. *Suicide Life Threat Behav, 13*, 147–154.

Haight BK. (1992). Long-term effects of structured life review process in homebound elderly subjects. *J Gerontol B Psychol Soc Sci, 47*, 312–315.

Hamerman D. (2010). Integrating aging into geriatric practice: An emerging orientation for health care. *J Am Geriatr Soc, 58*, 2024–2025.

Haney EM, O'Neil ME, Carson S, et al. (2012). *Suicide risk factors and risk assessment tools: A systematic review.* VA-ESP Project No. 05-225. Washington, DC: Department of Veterans Affairs.

Haney EM, Warden SJ. (2008). Skeletal effects of serotonin (5-hydroxytriptymine) transporter inhibition: Evidence from clinical studies. *J Musculoskelet Neuronal Interact, 8*, 133–145.

Hanlon JT, Boudreau RM, Roumani YF, et al. (2009). Number and dosage of central nervous system medications on recurrent falls in community elders: The Health, Aging, and Body Composition Study. *J Gerontol A Biol Sci Med Sci, 64*(4), 492–498.

Hanson AR, Scogin F. (2008). Older adults' acceptance of psychological, pharmacological and combination treatments for geriatric depression. *J Gerontol B Psychol Sci Soc Sci, 63*(4), P245–P248.

Harvey SB, Hotopf M, Øverland S, et al. (2010). Physical activity and common mental disorders. *Br J Psychiatry, 197*, 357–364.

Hay DP, Hay L, Blackwell B, et al. (1990). ECT and tardive dyskinesia. *J Geriatr Psychiatry Neurol, 3*(2), 106–109.

Hayward RD, Taylor WD, Smoski MJ, et al. (2013). Association of five-factor model personality domains and facets with presence, onset, and treatment outcomes of major depression in older adults. *Am J Geriatr Psychiatry, 21*, 88–96.

Hegel MT, Dietrich AJ, Seville JL, et al. (2004). Training residents in problem-solving treatment of depression: A pilot feasibility and impact study. *Fam Med, 36*, 204–208.

Hegerl U, Althaus D, Schmidtke A, et al. (2006). The alliance against depression: 2-year evaluation of a community-based intervention to reduce suicidality. *Psychol Med, 36*, 1225–1233.

Heisel M, Duberstein P, Talbot N, et al. (2009). Adapting interpersonal psychotherapy for older adults at risk for suicide: Preliminary findings. *Professional Psychology: Research and Practice, 40*, 156–164.

Hickie IB. (2011). Antidepressants in elderly people. *BMJ, 343*, d4660.

Hilty DM, Leamon MH, Lim RF, et al. (2006). Diagnosis and treatment of bipolar disorder in the primary care setting: A concise review. *Primary Psychiatry, 13*(7), 77–85.

Hirschfeld RMA. (2005). *Guideline watch: Practice guideline for the treatment of patients with bipolar disorder* (2nd ed.). Arlington, VA: American Psychiatric Association. Available online at *http://psychiatryonline.org/content.aspx?bookid=28&sectionid=1682557.*

Hoge CW, Castro CA. (2012). Preventing suicides in US service members and veterans. *JAMA, 308*(7), 671–672.

Huang KC, Lucas LF, Tsueda K, et al. (1989). Age-related changes in cardiovascular function associated with electroconvulsive therapy. *Convuls Ther, 5,* 17–25.

Hunkeler EM, Meresman JF, Hargreaves WA, et al. (2000). Efficacy of nurse telehealth care and peer support in augmenting treatment of depression in primary care. *Arch Fam Med, 9,* 700–708.

Husain MM, Rush AJ, Fink M, et al. (2004). Speed of response and remission in major depressive disorder with acute electroconvulsive therapy (ECT): A Consortium for Research in ECT (CORE) report. *J Clin Psychiatry, 65,* 485–491.

Jackson RD, LaCroix AZ, Gass M, et al. (2006). Calcium plus vitamin D supplementation and the risk of fractures. *N Engl J Med, 354*(7), 669–683.

Jayakody K, Gunadasa S, Hosker C. (2014). Exercise for anxiety disorders: Systematic review. *Br J Sports Med, 48*(3), 187–196.

Joo JH, Lenze EJ, Mulsant BH, et al. (2002). Risk factors for falls during treatment of late-life depression. *J Clin Psychiatry, 63,* 936–941.

Jorde R, Sneve M, Figenschau J, et al. (2008). Effects of vitamin D supplementation on symptoms of depression in overweight and obese subjects: Randomized double blind trial. *J Intern Med, 264*(6), 599–609.

Jorm AF, Christensen H, Griffiths KM. (2005). The impact of beyondblue: The national depression initiative on the Australian public's recognition of depression and beliefs about treatment. *Aust NZ J Psychiat, 39,* 248–254.

Kahana B, Kahana E, Harel Z. (1988). Coping with extreme stress. In JP Wilson, Z Harel, & B Kahana (Eds.), *Human adaptation to extreme stress: From the Holocaust to Viet Nam.* New York: Plenum Press.

Karasu TB. (1986). The specificity versus non specificity dilemma: Toward identifying therapeutic change agents. *Am J Psychiatry, 143,* 687–695

Karg K, Burmeister M, Sheddend K, et al. (2011, January 3). The serotonin transporter promoter variant (5-HTTLPR), stress, and depression meta-analysis revisited: Evidence of genetic moderation. *Arch Gen Psychiatry, 68*(5), 444–454.

Karp JF, Reynolds CF III. (2004). Pharmacotherapy of depression in the elderly: Achieving and maintaining optimal outcomes. *Primary Psychiatry, 11*(5), 37–46.

Katon WJ, Lin E, Russo J, et al. (2003). Increased medical costs of a population based sample of depressed elderly patients. *Arch Gen Psychiatry, 60,* 897–903.

Katon WJ, Lin EH, Von Korff M, et al. (2010). Collaborative care for patients with depression and chronic illnesses. *N Engl J Med, 363*(27), 2611–2620.

Katona C, Hansen T, Olsen CK. (2012). A randomized, double blind, placebo-controlled duloxetine-referenced, fixed dose study comparing the efficacy and safety of Lu AA21004 in elderly patients with major depressive disorder. *Int Clin Psychopharmacol, 27*(4), 215–223.

Katz I. (2012). Lessons learned from mental health enhancement and suicide prevention activities in the Veterans Health Administration. *Am J Public Health, 102*(Suppl. 1), S14–S16.

Kellner CH, Greenberg RM, Murrough JW, et al. (2012). ECT in treatment-resistant depression. *Am J Psychiatry, 169,* 1238–1244.

Kellner CH, Knapp RG, Petrides G, et al. (2006). Continuation electroconvulsive therapy vs pharmacotherapy for relapse prevention in major depression: A multisite study from the Consortium for Research in Electroconvulsive Therapy (CORE). *Arch Gen Psychiatry, 63,* 1337–1344.

Kendler KS, Gardner, MD, Prescott, CA. (2002). Toward a comprehensive developmental model for major depression in women. *Am J Psych, 159,* 1133–1145.

Kennedy GJ. (2000). *Geriatric mental health care: A treatment guide for health professionals.* New York: Guilford Press.

Kennedy GJ. (2005). Psychotherapies and other psychosocial interventions for depression in late life: Innovation through hybridization. *Primary Psychiatry, 12,* 16–20.

Kennedy GJ. (2006). The Sequenced Treatment Alternatives to Relieve Depression (STAR*D) studies: How applicable are the results for older adults? *Primary Psychiatry, 13*(11), 33–36.

Kennedy GJ. (2007). Exercise, aging and mental health. *Primary Psychiatry, 14*(4), 23–28.

Kennedy GJ. (2008). Bipolar disorder in late life: Depression. *Primary Psychiatry, 15*(3), 30–34.

Kennedy GJ. (2013). Depression and other mood disorders. In JT Pacala & GM Sullivan (Eds.), *Geriatrics review syllabus: A core curriculum in geriatric medicine* (8th ed., pp. 340–351). New York: American Geriatrics Society.

Kennedy GJ, Bader C, Beard JR, et al. (2014, March 16). *Why do older community residents affirm thoughts of "You would be better off dead or hurting yourself" from the Patient Health Questionnaire-9 (PHQ-9)?* Poster presented at the annual meeting of the American Association for Geriatric Psychiatry, Orlando, FL.

Kennedy GJ, Kastenschmidt E. (2010). Prevention of dementia and cognitive decline: Notes from the NIH-State-of-the- Science Conference. *Primary Psychiatry, 17*(7), 26–30.

Kennedy GJ, Kelman HR, Thomas C. (1990). Emergence of depressive symptoms in late life: The importance of declining health and increasing disability. *J Community Health, 15,* 93–104.

Kennedy GJ, Kelman HR, Thomas C. (1991). Persistence and remission of depressive symptoms in late life. *Am J Psychiatry, 148,* 174–178.

Kennedy GJ, Marcus P. (2005). Use of antidepressants in older patients with co-morbid medical conditions: Guidance from studies of depression in somatic illness. *Drugs Aging, 22*(4), 273–287.

King AC, Oman RF, Brassington GS, et al. (1997). Moderate intensity exercise and self-rated quality of sleep in older adults: A randomized controlled trial. *JAMA, 277,* 32–37.

King, AC, Pruitt LA, Phillips W, et al. (2000). Comparative effects of two physical activity programs on measured and perceived physical functioning and other health-related quality of life outcomes in older adults. *J Gerontol A Biol Sci Med Sci, 55*, M74–M83.

Knox KL, Conwell Y, Caine ED. (2004). If suicide is a public health problem, what are we doing to prevent it ? *Am J Public Health, 94*, 37–45.

Kobak K, Taylor L, Dottl S, et al. (1997). A computer-administered telephone interview to identify mental disorders. *JAMA, 278*, 905–910.

Korte J, Bohlmeijer ET, Cappeliez P, et al. (2011). Life review therapy for older adults with moderate depressive symptomatology: A pragmatic randomized controlled trial. *Psychol Med, 42*(6), 1163–1173.

Kramer AF, Hahn S, Cohen N, et al. (1999). Aging, fitness, and neurocognitive function. *Nature, 400*, 418–419.

Krause CA, Kunik ME, Stanley MA. (2007). Use of cognitive behavioral therapy in late-life psychiatric disorders. *Geriatrics, 62*, 21–26.

Krishnan KR, Doraiswamy PM, Clary CM. (2001). Clinical and treatment response characteristics of late-life depression associated with vascular disease: A pooled analysis of two multicenter trials with sertraline. *Prog Neuropsychopharmacol Biol Psychiatry, 25*(2), 347–361.

Krishnan KR, McDonald WM, Doraiswamy PM, et al. (1993). Neuroanatomical substrates of depression in the elderly. *Eur Arch Psychiatry Clin Neurosci, 243*(1), 41–46.

Krishnan KR, Taylor WD, McQuoid DR, et al. (2004). Clinical characteristics of magnetic resonance imaging-defined subcortical ischemic depression. *Biol Psychiatry, 55*(4), 390–397.

Kristal AR, Curry SJ, Shattuck AL, et al. (2000). A randomized trial of a tailored, self-help dietary intervention: The Puget Sound Eating Patterns study. *Prev Med, 31*(4), 380–389.

Kroenke K, Spitzer RL. (2002). The PHQ-9: A new depression diagnostic and severity measure. *Psychiatr Ann, 32*, 1–7.

Lakey B, Lutz CJ. (1996). Social support and preventive and therapeutic interventions. In GR Pierce, BR Sarason, & IG Sarason (Eds.), *Handbook of social support and the family* (pp. 435–465). New York, NY: Plenum Press.

Lamers F, Jonkers CC, Bosma H, et al. (2006). Effectiveness and cost-effectiveness of a minimal psychosocial intervention to reduce non-severe depression in chronically ill elderly patients: The design of a randomized controlled trial. *BMC Public Health, 6*, 161.

Lapierre S, Dubé M, Bouffard L, et al. (2007). Addressing suicidal ideations with the realization of meaningful personal goals. *Crisis, 28*, 16–25.

Lapierre S, Erlangsen A, Waern M, et al. (2011). A systematic review of elderly suicide prevention programs. *Crisis, 32*(2), 88–98.

Lavretsky H, Kumar A. (2002). Clinically significant non-major depression: Old concepts, new insights. *Am J Geriatr Psychiatry, 10*, 239–255.

Law LL, Barnett F, Yau MK, et al. (2014, March 11). Effects of combined cognitive and exercise interventions on cognition in older adults with and without cognitive impairment: A systematic review. *Ageing Res Rev, 15*, 61–75.

Lawton MP. (1994). Quality of life in Alzheimer disease. *Alzheimer Dis Assoc Disord, 8*(3), 138–150.

Lazarus LW, Sadavoy J. (1996). Individual psychotherapy. In J Sadavoy, LW Lazarus, & LF Jarvik (Eds.), *Comprehensive review of geriatric psychiatry-II* (2nd ed., pp. 819–850). Washington, DC: American Psychiatric Press.

Leverich GS, Altshuler LL, Frye MA, et al. (2006). Risk of switch on mood polarity to hypomania or mania in patients with bipolar depression during acute and continuation trials of venlafaxine, sertraline, and bupropion as adjuncts to mood stabilizers. *Am J Psychiatry, 162*(9), 232–239.

Lewinsohn PM. (1975). The behavioral study and treatment of depression. In M Hersen, RM Eisler, & PM Miller (Eds.), *Progress in behavior modification* (pp. 19–64). New York: Academic Press.

Li G, Mbuagbaw L, Samaan Z, et al. (2014). Efficacy of vitamin D supplementation in depression in adults: A systematic review. *J Clin Endocrinol Metab, 99*(3), 757–767.

Lichtman JH, Froelicher ES, Blumenthal JA, et al. (2014). Depression as a risk factor for poor prognosis among patients with acute coronary syndrome: Systematic review and recommendations. *Circulation.* Available at *http://circ.ahajournals.org/content/early/2014/02/24/CIR.0000000000000019.*

Light E, Niederhe G, Lebowitz BD (Eds.). (1994). *Stress effects on family caregivers of Alzheimer's patients.* New York: Springer.

Lisanby SH. (2007). Electroconvulsive therapy of depression. *N Engl J Med, 357,* 1939–1945.

Luoma JB, Martin CE, Pearson JL. (2002). Contact with mental health and primary care providers before suicide: A review of the evidence. *Am J Psychiatry, 159*(6), 909–916.

Lyketsos CG, Steinberg M, Tschanz JT, et al. (2001). Neuropsychiatric disturbance in Alzheimer's disease clusters into three groups: The Cache County Study. *Int J Geriatr Psychiatry, 16*(11), 1043–1053.

Lynch TR, Morse JQ, Mendelson T, et al. (2003). Dialectical behavior therapy for depressed older adults: A randomized pilot study. *Am J Geriatr Psychiatry, 11,* 33–45.

Lyness JM, Caine ED, King DA, et al. (2002). Depressive disorders and symptoms in older primary care patients: One-year outcomes. *Am J Geriatr Psychiatry, 10,* 275–282.

Lyness JM, Chapman BP, McGriff J, et al. (2009). One-year outcomes of minor and subsyndromal depression in older primary care patients. *Int Psychogeriatr, 21*(1), 60–68.

Lyness JM, Heo M, Datto CJ, et al. (2006). Outcomes of minor and subsyndromal depression among elderly patients in primary care settings. *Ann Intern Med, 144,* 496–504.

Lyness JM, Kim J, Tang W, et al. (2007). The clinical significance of subsyndromal depression in older primary care patients. *Am J Geriatr Psychiatry, 15,* 214–223.

Lyness JM, King DA, Cox C, et al. (1999). The importance of subsyndromal depression in older primary care patients: prevalence and associated functional disability. *J Am Geriatr Soc, 47*(6), 647–652.

Malberg JE, Eisch AJ, Nestler EJ, et al. (2000). Chronic antidepressant treatment increases neurogenesis in adult rat hippocampus. *J Neurosci, 20*, 9104–9110.

Malmstrom TK, Wolinsky FD, Andresen EM, et al. (2005). Cognitive ability and physical performance in middle-aged African Americans. *J Am Geriatr Soc, 53*, 997–1001.

Mamdani MM, Herrman N, Austin P. (1999). Prevalence of antidepressant use among older people: Population-based observations. *J Am Geriatr Soc, 47*, 1350–1353.

Mamdani MM, Parikh SV, Austin PC, et al. (2000). Use of antidepressants among elderly subjects: Trends and contributing factors. *Am J Psychiatry, 157*, 238–230.

Mann JJ, Apter A, Bertolote J, et al. (2005). Suicide prevention strategies: A systematic review. *JAMA, 294*, 2064–2074.

Manson JE, Hu FB, Rich-Edwards JW, et al. (1999). A prospective study of walking as compared with vigorous exercise in the prevention of coronary heart disease in women. *N Engl J Med, 341*, 650–658.

Martenson R. (2008). *A life worth living: A doctor's reflections on illness in a high-tech era.* New York: Farrar, Straus & Giroux.

Martire LM, Lustig AP, Schulz R, et al. (2004). Is it beneficial to involve a family member? A meta-analysis of psychosocial intervention for chronic illness. *Health Psychology, 23*, 599–611.

Mast BT, Yochim B, MacNeill SE, et al. (2004). Risk factors for geriatric depression: The importance of executive functioning within the vascular depression hypothesis. *J Gerontol A Biol Sci Med Sci, 59*(12), 1290–1294.

Mathers CD, Loncar D. (2006). Projections of global mortality and burden of disease from 2002 to 2030. *PLoS Med, 3*(11), e44.

May HT, Bair TL, Lappé DL, et al. (2010). Association of vitamin D levels with incident depression among a general cardiovascular population. *Am Heart J, 159*(6), 1037–1043.

Mayer-Davis EJ, D'Agostino R Jr, Karter AJ, et al. (1998). Intensity and amount of physical activity in relation to insulin sensitivity: The Insulin Resistance Atherosclerosis Study. *JAMA, 279*, 669–674.

Mayo Clinic Staff. (2010). Mediterranean diet: Choose this heart-healthy option. Retrieved October 25, 2010, from *www.mayoclinic.org/healthy-living/nutrition-and-health-eating/in-depth/mediterranean-diet/art-20047801.*

McDonald WM, Krishnan KRR, Doraiswamy PM, et al. (1991). The occurrence of subcortical hyperintensities in patients with mania. *Psychiatry Res, 40*, 211–220.

McGrath PJ, Stewart JW, Fava M, et al. (2006). Tranylcypromine versus venlafaxine plus mirtazapine following three failed antidepressant medication trials for depression: A STAR*D report. *Am J Psychiatry, 163*, 1531–1541.

McKeown RE, Cuffe SP, Schulz RM. (2006). US suicide rates by age group, 1970–2002: An examination of recent trends. *Am J Public Health, 96*, 1744–1751.

McLennan SN, Mathias JL. (2010). The depression-executive dysfunction (DED) syndrome and response to antidepressants: A meta-analytic review. *Int J Geriatr Psychiatry, 25*(10), 933–944.

Mental disorders and general practice. (1906). *JAMA, 46,* 1700–1701. (Reprinted by *JAMA* in 2006)

Mental Health Parity and Addiction Equity Act of 2008, Pub. L. No. 110-343 (2008), 122 Stat. 3765.

MetLife Mature Market Institute and the National Alliance for Caregiving. (2006). *The MetLife caregiving cost study: Productivity losses to U.S. business.* Available at *www.metlife.com/mmi/research/working-caregiver-employer-health-care-costs.html#findings.*

Meyers BS, Flint, AJ, Rothschild, AJ, et al. (2009). A double-blind randomized controlled trial of olanzapine plus sertraline versus olanzapine plus placebo for psychotic depression. *Arch Gen Psychiatry, 66*(8), 838–847.

Meyers BS, Klimstra SA, Gabriele M, et al. (2001). Continuation treatment of delusional depression in older adults. *Am J Psychiatry, 9*(4), 415–422.

Meyers BS, Peasly-Miklus C, Flint AJ, et al. (2006). Methodological issues in designing a randomized controlled trial for psychotic depression: The STOP-PD study. *Psychiatr Ann, 36*(1), 57–64.

Mikami K, Jorge RE, Moser DJ, et al. (2014, January 23). Prevention of post-stroke generalized anxiety disorder, using escitalopram or problem-solving therapy. *J Neuropsychiatry Clin Neurosci.*

Miklowitz DJ, George EL, Richards JA, et al. (2003). A randomized study of family-focused psychoeducation and pharmacotherapy in the outpatient management of bipolar disorder. *Arch Gen Psychiatry, 60,* 904–912.

Miklowitz DJ, Otto MW, Frank E, et al. (2007a). Psychosocial treatments for bipolar depression: A 1-year randomized trial from the systematic treatment enhancement program. *Arch Gen Psychiatry, 64,* 419–426.

Miklowitz GJ, Otto MW, Frank E, et al. (2007b). Intensive psychosocial intervention enhances functioning in patients with bipolar depression: Results from a 9-month randomized controlled trial. *Am J Psychiatry, 164*(9), 1340–1347.

Miller M, Azrael D, Barber C. (2012). Suicide mortality in the United States: The importance of attending to method in understanding population-level disparities in the burden of suicide. *Ann Rev Public Health, 33,* 393–408.

Miller MD, Silberman RI. (1996). Using interpersonal psychotherapy with depressed elderly. In SH Zarit & BG Knight (Eds.), *A guide to psychotherapy and aging* (pp. 83–100). New York: American Psychological Association.

Miller MD, Cornes C, Frank E, et al. (2001). Interpersonal psychotherapy for late-life depression: Past, present and future. *J Psychotherapy Practice and Research, 10,* 231–238.

Milstein G, Kennedy GJ, Bruce ML, et al. (2005). The clergy's role in reducing stigma: A bi-lingual study of elder patients' views. *World Psychiatry, 4*(S1), 28–34.

Mitchell AJ, Vaze A, Rao S. (2009). Clinical diagnosis of depression in primary care: A meta-analysis. *Lancet, 374,* 609–619.

Mitchell SR, Wilhelm K, Parker G. (2001). The clinical features of bipolar depression: A comparison with matched major depressive disorder patients. *J Clin Psychiatry, 62,* 212–216.

Mittelman MS, Ferris SH, Shulman E, et al. (1995). A comprehensive support program: Effect on depression in spouse-caregivers of AD patients. *Gerontologist, 35,* 792–802.

Mittelman MS, Roth DL, Clay OJ, et al. (2007). Preserving health of Alzheimer caregivers: Impact of a spouse caregiver intervention. *Am J Geriatr Psychiatry, 15*(9), 780–789.

Mittelman MS, Brodaty H, Wallen AS, et al. (2008). A three-country randomized controlled trial of a psychosocial intervention for caregivers combined with pharmacological treatment for patients with Alzheimer disease: Effect on caregiver depression. *Am J Geriatr Psychiatry, 16*(11), 893–904.

Mohlman J, Bryant C, Lenze EJ, et al. (2012). Improving recognition of late life anxiety disorders in *Diagnostic and Statistical Manual of Mental Disorders, fifth edition:* Observations and recommendations of the Advisory Committee to the Lifespan Disorders Work Group. *Int J Geriatr Psychiatry, 27*(6), 549–556.

Mohr DC, Ho J, Duffecy J, et al. (2012). Effect of telephone-administered vs face-to-face cognitive behavioral therapy on adherence to therapy and depression outcomes among primary care patients. *JAMA, 307*(21), 2278–2285.

Mohr DC, Stacey SL, Julian L, et al. (2005). Telephone-administered psychotherapy for depression. *Arch Gen Psychiatry, 62,* 1007–1014.

Mojtabai R. (2014). Diagnosing depression in older adults in primary care. *N Eng J Med, 370*(13), 1180–1182.

Morimoto SS, Gunning FM, Murphy CF, et al. (2011). Executive function and short-term remission of geriatric depression: The role of semantic strategy. *Am J Geriatr Psychiatry, 19,* 115–122.

Mourilhe P, Stokes PE. (1998). Risk and benefits of selective serotonergic reuptake inhibitors in the treatment of depression. *Drug Saf, 18,* 57–82.

Murphy SL, Xu JQ, Kochanek KD. (2013). Deaths: Final data for 2010. *National Vital Statistics Reports, 61*(4), 1–117. Hyattsville, MD: National Center for Health Statistics.

Mulsant BH, Alexopoulos GS, Reynolds CF Jr, et al. (2001a). Pharmacologic treatment of older primary care patients: The PROSPECT algorithm. *J Geri Psychiatry, 16,* 585–592.

Mulsant BH, Houck PR, Gildengers AG, et al. (2006). What is the optimal duration of a short-term antidepressant trial when treating geriatric depression? *J Clin Psychopharmacol, 26*(2), 113–120.

Mulsant BH, Sweet RA, Rosen J, et al. (2001b). A double-blind, randomized comparison of nortriptyline plus perphenazine versus nortriptyline plus placebo in the treatment of psychotic depression. *J Clin Psychiatry, 62*(8), 597–604.

Mulsant BH, Blumberger DM, Ismail Z, et al. (2014). A systematic approach to pharmacotherapy for geriatric depression. *Clin Geriatr Med, 30,* 517–534.

Murphy FC, Sahakian BJ, Rubinsztein JS, et al. (1999). Emotional bias and inhibitory control processes in mania and depression. *Psychol Medicine, 29,* 1307–1321.

Musselman D, Lawson D, Gumnick J, et al. (2001). Paroxetine for the prevention of depression induced by high-dose interferon alfa. *N Engl J Med, 344,* 961–966.

National Heart, Lung and Blood Institute. (1998). Clinical guidelines on the identification, evaluation, and treatment of overweight and obesity in adults—The evidence report. National Institutes of Health. *Obesity Research, 6,* 51S-209S.

National Institute on Aging. (1999). *Exercise: A guide from the national institute on aging.* Public Information Office, National Institute on Aging, NIH Publication No. 99-4258.

National Institute for Health and Clinical Excellence. (2006). Computerised cognitive behaviour therapy for depression and anxiety: Review of technology appraisal 51. Retrieved April 4, 2012, from *www.nice.org.uk/TA097.*

National Institute for Health and Clinical Excellence. (2009). Guidelines for treatment and management of depression in adults. Available at *www.nice.org.uk/nicemedia/live/12329/45888/45888.pdf.*

National Research Council. (2000). *Dietary reference intakes: Applications in dietary assessment.* Washington, DC: National Academies Press.

Nemeroff CB, Evans DL, Gyulai L, et al. (2001). Double-blind, placebo controlled comparison of imipramine and paroxetine in the treatment of bipolar depression. *Am J Psychiatry, 158,* 906–912.

Nesheim MC, Yaktine AL (Eds.). (2007). *Seafood choices: Balancing benefits and risks.* Washington, DC: National Academies Press. Retrieved November 30, 2010, from *www.nap.edu/catalog/11762.html.*

New York Times. (2013, February 15). *Suicide made easier* [Editorial], p. A26.

Nezu AM, Nezu CM, Perri MG. (1989). *Problem solving therapy for depression: Theory, research, and clinical guidelines.* Oxford, UK: Wiley.

Nierenberg AA, Fava M, Trivedi MH, et al. (2006a). A comparison of lithium and T3 augmentation following two failed medication treatments for depression: A STAR*D report. *Am J Psychiatry, 163,* 1519–1530.

Nierenberg AA, Ostacher MJ, Calabrese JR, et al. (2006b). Treatment-resistant bipolar depression: A STEP-BD equipoise randomized effectiveness trial of antidepressant augmentation with lamotrigine, inositol, or risperidone. *Am J Psychiatry, 163*(2), 210–216.

Niederehe G. (1996). Psychosocial treatments with older depressed adults. *Am J Geriatr Psychiatry, 4*(Suppl. 1), S66–S78.

Nolan M, Keady J, Grant G. (1995). Developing a typology of family care: Implications for nurses and other service providers. *J Adv Nurs, 21*(2), 256–265.

Novick P (1999). *The Holocaust in American life.* New York: Houghton Mifflin.

O'Connor E, Whitlock, EP, Gaynes B, et al. (2009). *Screening for depression in adults and older adults in primary care: An updated systematic review.* AHRQ Publication No. 10-05143-EF-1. Rockville, MD: Agency for Healthcare Research and Quality.

O'Connor MK, Knapp R, Husain M, et al. (2001). The influence of age on the response of major depression to electroconvulsive therapy: A C.O.R.E. report. *Am J Geri Psychiatry, 9,* 382–90.

Oliffe JL, Rasmussen B, Bottorff JL, et al. (2013). Masculinities, work, and retirement among older men who experience depression. *Qual Health Res,* 23(12), 1626–1637.

Olin JT, Schneider L, Katz I, et al. (2002). Provisional diagnostic criteria for depression of Alzheimer's disease. *Am J Geriatr Psychiatry, 10,* 125–128.

Oslin DW. (2005). Treatment of late-life depression complicated by alcohol dependence. *Am J Geriatric Psychiatry, 13,* 491–500.

Owens et al. (2007). *Care of adults with mental health and substance abuse disorders in U.S. Community Hospitals, 2004.* AHRQ Publication No. 07–0008. Rockville, MD: Agency for Healthcare Research and Quality.

Oxman TE. (2003). *Re-engineering systems for primary care treatment of depression: The respect depression care process supervising psychiatrist manual.* Hanover, NH: Trustees of Dartmouth College.

Oxman TE, Barrett JE, Sengupta A, et al. (2001). Status of minor depression or dysthymia in primary care following a randomized controlled treatment. *Gen Hosp Psychiatry, 23,* 301–310.

Oxman TE, Hull JG. (1997). Social support, depression, and activities of daily living in older heart surgery patients. *J Gerontol B Psychol Sci Soc Sci, 52,* P1–P14.

Parker G, Roy K, Hadzi-Pavlovic D, et al. (1992). Psychotic (delusional) depression: A meta-analysis of physical treatments. *J Affect Disord, 24,* 17–24.

Patel V, Shekar S. (2014). Transforming lives, enhancing communities: Innovations in global health. *N Engl J Med, 370*(6), 498–501.

Paykel ES, Tylee A, Wright A, et al. (1997). The Defeat Depression Campaign: Psychiatry in the public arena. *Am J Psychiatry, 154,* 59–65.

Pearlman LA, Wortman CB, Feuer CA, et al. (2014). *Treating traumatic bereavement: A practitioner's guide.* New York: Guilford Press

Perlis RH, Ostacher MJ, Patel JK, et al. (2006a). Predictors of recurrence in bipolar disorder: Primary outcomes from the systematic Treatment Enhancement Program for Bipolar Disorders (STEP-BD). *Am J Psychiatry, 163*(2), 217–224.

Perlis RH, Weige JA, Vornik LA, et al. (2006b). Atypical antipsychotics in the treatment of mania: A meta-analysis of randomized, placebo-controlled trials. *J Clin Psychiatry, 67*(4), 509–516.

Petrides G, Fink M, Husain MM, et al. (2001). ECT remission rates in psychotic versus nonpsychotic depressed patients: A report from CORE. *J ECT, 17*(4), 244–253.

Phillips KA. (2004). Psychosis in body dysmorphic disorder. *J Psychiatr Res, 38*(1), 63–72.

Pickett YR, Ghosh S, Rohs A, et al. (2014a). Healthcare use among older primary care patients with minor depression. *Am J Geriatr Psychiatry, 22*(2), 207–210.

Pickett YR, Kennedy GJ, Freeman K, et al. (2014b). The effect of telephone-facilitated depression care on older, medically ill patients. *J Behav Health Serv Res, 41*(1), 90–96.

Pierce GR, Sarason IG, & Sarason BR. (1991). General and relationship based perceptions of support: Are two constructs better than one? *J Pers Soc Psychol, 61,* 1028–1039.

Pinquart M, Duberstein P, Lyness JM. (2006). Treatments for later-life depressive conditions: A meta-analytic comparison of pharmacotherapy and psychotherapy. *Am J Psychiatry, 163*(9), 1493–1501.

Plutchik R, Botsis AJ, Weiner MB, et al. (1996). Clinical measurement of suicidality and coping in late life: A theory of countervailing forces. In GJ Kennedy (Ed.), *Suicide and depression in late life* (pp. 83–102). New York: Wiley.

Podgorski CA, Langford L, Pearson JL, et al. (2010). Suicide prevention for older adults in residential communities: Implications for policy and practice.

PLoS Med, 7(5), e1000254.

Porsteinsson AP, Drye LT, Pollock BG, et al. (2014). Effect of citalopram on agitation in Alzheimer disease: The CitAD randomized clinical trial. *JAMA, 311*(7), 682–691.

President's New Freedom Commission on Mental Health. (2003). *Achieving the Promise: Transforming Mental Health Care in America.* Retrieved March 25, 2009, *from www.mentalhealthcommission.gov/reports/reports.htm.*

Prigerson HG, Monk TH, Reynolds CF III, et al. (1995/1996). Lifestyle regularity and activity level as protective factors against bereavement-related depression in late life. *Depression, 3,* 297–302.

Prudic J, Olfson M, Marcus SC, et al. (2004). Effectiveness of electroconvulsive therapy in community settings. *Biol Psychiatry, 55*(3), 301–312.

Prudic J, Peyser S, Sackeim HA. (2000). Subjective memory complaints: A review of patient self-assessment of memory after electroconvulsive therapy. *J ECT 16,* 121–132.

Pugh KG, Kiely DK, Milberg WP, et al. (2003). Selective impairment of frontal-executive cognitive function in African Americans with cardiovascular risk factors. *J Am Geriatr Soc, 51,* 1439–1444.

Raue PJ, Brown EL, Meyers BS, et al. (2006). Does every allusion to possible suicide require the same response? *J Fam Pract, 55,* 605–612.

Reifler BV, Cox GB, Hanley RJ. (1981). Problems of mentally ill elderly as perceived by patients, families, and clinicians. *Gerontologist, 21*(2), 165–170.

Resnick B. (2003). Exercise for older adults: What to prescribe and how to motivate. *Caring for the Ages, 4*(1), 8–12.

Resnick B, Spellbring A. (2000). Who wants to live to be 100? Understanding what motivates older adults to exercise. *J Gerontol Nurs, 26,* 34–42.

Ressler KJ, Mayberg HS. (2007). Targeting abnormal neural circuits in mood and anxiety disorders: From the laboratory to the clinic. *Nature Neuroscience, 10*(9), 1116–1124.

Revest JM, Dupret D, Koehl M, et al. (2009). Adult hippocampal neurogenesis is involved in anxiety-related behaviors. *Mol Psychiatry, 14,* 959–967.

Reynolds CF III. (2008). Preventing depression in old age: It's time? *Am J Geriatr Psychiatry, 16*(6), 433–434.

Reynolds CF III, Butters MA, Lopez O, et al. (2011). Maintenance treatment of depression in old age: A randomized, double-blind, placebo-controlled evaluation of the efficacy and safety of donepezil combined with antidepressant pharmacotherapy. *Arch Gen Psychiatry, 68*(1), 51–60.

Reynolds CF III, Dew MA, Martire LM, et al. (2010). Treating depression to remission in older adults: A controlled evaluation of combined interpersonal psychotherapy versus escitalopram with depression care management. *Int J Geriatr Psychiatry, 25*, 1134–1141.

Reynolds CF III, Dew MA, Pollock BJ, et al. (2006). Maintenance treatment of major depression in old age. *N Engl J Med, 354*, 1130–1138.

Reynolds CF III, Miller MD, Pasternak RE, et al. (1999). Treatment of bereavement-related major depressive episodes in later life: A randomized, double-blind, placebo controlled study of acute and continuation treatment with nortriptyline and interpersonal psychotherapy. *Am J Psychiatry, 156*, 202–208.

Ricker JH, Axelrod BN. (1994). Analysis of an oral paradigm for the Trail Making Test. *Assessment, 1*(1), 47–52.

Riddick CC, Cohen-Mansfield J, Fleshner E, et al. (1992). Caregiver adaptations to having a relative with dementia admitted to a nursing home. *J Gerontol Soc Work, 19*, 51–76.

Robinson GK. (1990). The psychiatric component of long-term care models. In BS Fogel, A Furino, & GL Gottlieb (Eds.), *Mental health policy for older Americans: Protecting minds at risk* (pp. 157–178). Washington DC: American Psychiatric Press.

Robinson RG, Jorge RE, Moser DJ, et al. (2008). Escitalopram and problem-solving therapy for prevention of post-stroke depression: A randomized controlled trial. JAMA, *299*(20), 2391–2400.

Rocha Araujo DM, Vilarim MM, Nardi AE. (2010). What is the effectiveness of the use of polyunsaturated fatty acid omega-3 in the treatment of depression? *Expert Rev Neurother, 10*(7), 1117–1129.

Rockett HR, Colditz GA. (1997). Assessing diets of children and adolescents. *Am J Clin Nutr, 65*(4), 1116–1122.

Rodin J, Langer EJ. (1977). Long-term effects of a control-relevant intervention with institutionalized aged. *J Pers Soc Psychol, 35*, 897–902.

Rondanelli M, Giacosa A, Opizzi A, et al. (2010). Effect of omega-3 fatty acids supplementation on depressive symptoms and on health-related quality of life in the treatment of elderly women with depression: A double-blind, placebo-controlled, randomized clinical trial. *J Am Coll Nutr, 29*(1), 55–64.

Roose SP, Sackeim HA. (2002). Clinical trials in late-life depression: Revisited. *Am J Geriatr Psychiatry, 10*, 503–505.

Rose JM, DelMaestro SG. (1990). Separation–individuation conflict as a model for understanding distressed caregivers: Psychodynamic and cognitive case studies. *Gerontologist, 30*(5), 693–697

Rosen CJ. (2009). Serotonin rising: The bone, brain, bowel connection. *N Engl J Med, 360*, 957–959.

Rosen J, Rogers JC, Marin RS, et al. (1997). Control-relevant intervention in the treatment of minor and major depression in a long-term care facility. *Am J Geriatr Psychiatry, 5*, 247–257.

Rothschild AJ, Mulsant BH, Meyers BS, et al. (2006). Challenges in differentiating and diagnosing psychotic depression. *Psychiatr Ann, 36*(1), 40–46.

Rovner B, Casten R. (2008). Preventing late-life depression in age-related macular degeneration. *Am J Geriatr, 16,* 454–459.

Rowe JW, Kahn RL. (1998). *Successful aging.* New York: Pantheon Books.

Royall DR, Cordes JA, Román G, et al. (2009). Sertraline improves executive function in patients with vascular cognitive impairment. *J Neuropsychiatry Clin Neurosci, 21*(4), 445–454.

Rush AJ, Beck AT. (1978). Cognitive therapy of depression and suicide. *Am J Psychother, 32*(2), 201–219.

Rush AJ, Trivedi M, Fava M. (2003). Depression IV: STAR*D treatment trial for depression. *Am J Psychiatry, 160*(2), 237.

Rush AJ, Trivedi MH, Wisniewski SR, et al. (2006). Bupropion-SR, sertraline, or venlafaxine-XR after failure of SSRIs for depression. *N Engl J Med, 354,* 1231–1242.

Rutz W, von Knorring L, Pihlgren H, et al. (1995). An educational project on depression and its consequences: Is the frequency of major depression among Swedish men under-rated, resulting in high suicidality? *Primary Care Psychiatry, 1,* 59–63.

Sachdev PS, Parslow RA, Lux O, et al. (2005). Relationship of homocysteine, folic acid and vitamin B12 with depression in a middle-aged community sample. *Psychol Med, 35*(4), 529–538.

Sachs GS, Nierenberg AA, Calabrese JR, et al. (2007). Effectiveness of adjunctive antidepressant treatment for bipolar depression. *N Engl J Med, 356*(17), 1711–1722.

Sackeim HA, Dillingham EM, Prudic J, et al. (2009). Effect of concomitant pharmacotherapy on electroconvulsive therapy outcomes: Short-term efficacy and adverse effects. *Arch Gen Psychiatry, 66*(7), 729–737.

Sackeim HA, Haskett RF, Mulsant BH, et al. (2001). Continuation pharmacotherapy in the prevention of relapse following electroconvulsive therapy: A randomized controlled trial. *JAMA, 285*(10), 1299–1307.

Sackeim HA, Prudic J. (2005). Length of ECT course in bipolar and unipolar depression. *J ECT, 21,*195–197.

Sackeim HA, Prudic J, Devanand DP, et al. (1993). Effects of stimulus intensity and electrode placement on the efficacy and cognitive effects of electroconvulsive therapy. *N Engl J Med, 328*(12), 839–846.

Sackeim HA, Prudic J, Fuller RB, et al. (2007). The cognitive effects of electroconvulsive therapy in community settings. *Neuropsychopharmacology, 32*(1), 244–254.

Sahay A, Hen R. (2007). Adult hippocampal neurogenesis in depression. *Nat Neurosci, 10*(9), 1110–1115. Review.

Sajatovic M, Blow FC, Ignacio RV, et al. (2005). New-onset bipolar disorder in later life. *Am J Geriatr Psychiatry, 13,* 282–289.

Sakauye K, Streim J, Kennedy GJ, et al. (2009). Disaster preparedness for older Americans: Critical issues for the preservation of mental health. *Am J Geriatr Psychiatry, 17*(12), 916–924.

Salzman C. (2001). *Psychiatric medications for older adults.* New York: Guilford Press.

Samuels BA, Hen R. (2001). Neurogenesis and affective disorders. *Eur J Neurosci, 33,* 1152–1159.

Samus QM, Johnston D, Black BS, et al. (2014). A multidimensional home-based care coordination intervention for elders with memory disorders: The Maximizing Independence at Home (MIND) pilot randomized trial. *Am J Geriatr Psychiatry, 22*(4), 398–414.

Sánchez-Villegas A, Delgado-Rodríguez M, Alonso A, Schlatter J, et al. (2009). Association of the Mediterranean dietary pattern with the incidence of depression: The Seguimiento Universidad de Navarra/University of Navarra Follow-up (SUN) Cohort. *Arch Gen Psychiatry, 66*(10), 1090–1098.

Stanislaw CA, Pine DS, Quinn KJ, et al. (2010). Developing constructs for psychopathology research: Research domain criteria. *J Abnorm Psychol, 119*(4), 631–639.

Santarelli L, Saxe M, Gross C, et al. (2003). Requirement of hippocampal neurogenesis for the behavioral effects of antidepressants. *Science, 301,* 805–809.

Sarason BR, Pierce GR, & Sarason IG. (1990). Social support: The sense of acceptance and the role of relationships. In BR Sarason, IG Sarason, & GR Pierce (Eds.), *Social support: An interactional view* (pp. 97–128). New York: Wiley.

Sato T. (2005). The Eysenck Personality Questionnaire Brief Version: Factor structure and reliability. *J Psychol, 139*(6), 545–552.

Sattin R, Easley KA, Wolf SL, et al. (2005). Reduction in fear of falling through intense tai chi exercise training in older, transitionally frail adults. *J Am Geriatr Soc, 53,* 1168–1178.

Saxena S, Thornicroft G, Knapp M, et al. (2007). Resources for mental health: Scarcity, inequity, and inefficiency. *Lancet, 370,* 878–889.

Schoevers RA, Beekman ATF, Deeg DJH, et al. (2003). The natural history of late-life depression: Results from the Amsterdam Study of the Elderly (AMSTEL). *J Affect Disord, 76,* 5–14.

Schoevers RA, Smit F, Deeg DJ, et al. (2006). Prevention of late-life depression in primary care: Do we know where to begin? *Am J Psychiatry, 163*(9), 1611–1621.

Schulz R. (1976). Effects of control and predictability on the physical and psychological well-being of the institutionalized aged. *J Pers Soc Psychol, 33,* 563–573.

Scogin F, McElreath L. (1994). Efficacy of psychosocial treatments for geriatric depression: A quantitative review. *J Consult Clin Psychol, 62,* 69–74.

Scogin F, Welsh D, Hanson A, et al. (2005). Evidence-based psychotherapies for depression in older adults. *Clin Psychol Sci Pract, 12,* 222–237.

Seeman TE, et al. (1995). Behavioral and psychosocial predictors of physical performance: MacArthur studies of successful aging. *J Gerontol A Biol Sci Med Sci,* 177–193.

Semple SJ. (1992). Conflict in Alzheimer's caregiving families: Its dimensions and consequences. *Gerontologist, 32,* 648–655.

Serby M. (2001). Manic reactions to ECT. *Am J Geriatr Psychiatry, 9,* 180.

Shear K. (2003). *Traumatic grief: Guidebook for enhanced services providers.* Pittsburgh: University of Pittsburgh,

Shear K, Frank E, Houck PR, et al. (2005). Treatment of complicated grief: A randomized controlled trial. *JAMA, 293,* 2601–2608.

Shear MK, Mulhare E. (2008). Complicated grief. *Psychiatr Ann, 38*(10), 662–670.

Sheline YI, Disabato BM, Hranilovich J, et al. (2012). Treatment course with antidepressant therapy in late-life depression. *Am J Psychiatry, 169,* 1185–1193.

Shelton RC, Hollon SD, Wisniewski SR, et al. (2009). Factors associated with concomitant psychotropic drug use in the treatment of major depression: A STAR*D report. *CNS Spectrums, 14*(9), 487–498.

Shepherd J, Cobbe SM, Ford I, et al. (1995). Prevention of coronary heart disease with pravastatin in men with hypercholesterolemia: West of Scotland Coronary Prevention Study Group. *N Engl J Med, 333*(20), 1301–1307.

Shuchter SR, Zisook S. (1993) The course of normal grief. In MS Stroebe & RO Hansson (Eds.), *Handbook of bereavement: Theory, research, and intervention* (pp. 23–43). Cambridge, UK: Cambridge University Press.

Shulman KI. (2010). Lithium for older adults with bipolar disorder: Should it still be considered a first-line agent? *Drugs Aging, 27*(8), 607–615.

Singh NA, Clementws KM, Fiatarone MA. (1997). A randomized trial of progressive resistance training in depressed elders. *J Gerontol A Biol Sci Med Sci, 52,* M27–M35.

Singh NA, Stavrinos TM, Scarbeck Y, et al. (2005). A randomized trial of high versus low intensity weight training versus general practitioner care for clinical depression in older adults. *J Gerontol A Biol Sci Med Sci, 60,* 768–776.

Singh-Manoux A, Hillsdon M, Brunner E, et al. (2005). Effects of physical activity on cognitive functioning in middle age: Evidence from the Whitehall II Prospective Cohort Study. *Am J Public Health, 95,* 2252–2258.

Sirey, JA, Bruce, ML, Alexopoulos, GS. (2005). The treatment initiation program: An intervention to improve depression outcomes in older adults. *Am J Psychiatry, 162,* 184–186.

Skarupski KA, Tangney C, Li H, et al. (2010). Longitudinal association of vitamin B-6, folate, and vitamin B-12 with depressive symptoms among older adults over time. *Am J Clin Nutr, 92*(2), 330–335.

Skultety KM, Zeiss A. (2006). The treatment of depression in older adults in the primary care setting: An evidence-based review. *Health Psychology, 25,* 665–674.

Smit F, Ederveen A, Cuijpers P, et al. (2006). Opportunities for cost-effective prevention of late-life depression: An epidemiological approach. *Arch Gen Psychiatry, 63*(3), 290–296.

Smits F, Smits N, Schoevers R, et al. (2008). An epidemiological approach to depression prevention in old age. *Am J Geriatr Psychiatry, 16*(6), 444–453.

Sneed JR, Culang ME, Keilp JG, et al. (2010). Antidepressant medication and executive dysfunction: A deleterious interaction in late-life depression. *Am J Geriatr Psychiatry, 18*, 128–135.

Song C, Wang H. (2011, April 29). Cytokines mediated inflammation and decreased neurogenesis in animal models of depression. *Prog Neuropsychopharmacol Biol Psychiatry, 35*(3), 760–768.

Souberbielle JC, Body JJ, Lappe JM, et al. (2010). Vitamin D and musculoskeletal health, cardiovascular disease, autoimmunity and cancer: Recommendations for clinical practice. *Autoimmun Rev, 9*(11), 709–715.

Springate BA, Tremont G. (2014). Dimensions of caregiver burden in dementia: impact of demographic, mood, and care recipient variables. *Am J Geriatr Psychiatry, 22*(3), 294–300.

Spitzer RL, Kroenke K, Williams JB, et al. (1995). Health related quality of life in primary care patients with mental disorders: Results from the PRIME-MD 1000 study. *JAMA, 274*, 1511–1517.

Spitzer RL, Kroenke K, Williams JB. (1999). Validation and utility of a self-report version of PRIME-MD: The PHQ primary care study. *JAMA, 282*, 1737–1744.

Spreen DD, Benton AL (1977). *Manual of instructions for the Neurosensory Center Comprehensive Examination for Aphasia.* Victoria, BC, Canada, University of Victoria.

Stahl SM, Pradko JF, Haight BR, et al. (2004). A review of the neuropharmacology of bupropion, a dual norepinephrine and dopamine reuptake inhibitor. *Prim Care Companion J Clin Psychiatry, 6*, 159–166.

Steffens DC, McQuoid DR, Krishnan RR. (2002). The Duke Somatic Algorithm for Geriatric Depression (STAGED) approach. *Psychopharmacology Bull, 36*(2), 58–68.

Steffens DC, Skoog I, Norton MC, et al. (2000). Prevalence of depression and its treatment in an elderly population: The Cache County study. *Arch Gen Psychiatry, 57*, 601–607.

Stewart JC, Perkins AJ, Callahan CM. (2014). Effect of collaborative care for depression on risk of cardiovascular events: Data from the IMPACT randomized controlled trial. *Psychosom Med, 76*(1), 29–37.

Stofan JR, DiPietro L, Davis D, et al. (1998). Physical activity patterns associated with cardiorespiratory fitness and reduced mortality: The Aerobics Fitness Center Longitudinal Study. *Am J Public Health, 88*, 1807–1813.

Strakowski SM. (2007). Approaching the challenge of bipolar depression: Results from STEP-BD. *Am J Psychiatry, 164*, 1301–1303.

Strohle A, Feller C, Onken M, et al. (2005). The acute anti-panic activity of aerobic exercise. *Am J Psychiatry, 162*, 2376–2378.

Swinburn, BA, Walter LG, Arroll B, et al. (1998). The green prescription study: A randomized controlled trial of written exercise advice provided by general practitioners. *Am J Public Health, 88*, 288–291.

Szanto K, Mulsant BH, Houck PR, et al. (2001). Treatment outcome in suicidal vs. non-suicidal elderly patients. *Am J Geriatr Psychiatry, 9*(3), 261–268.

Szanto K, Mulsant BH, Houck PR, et al. (2007). Emergence, persistence, and resolution of suicidal ideation during treatment of depression in old age. *J Affect Disord, 98*(1–2), 153–161.

Szanto K, Reynolds CE III, Frank E, et al. (1996). Suicide in elderly depressed patients: Is active vs. passive suicidal ideation a clinically valid distinction? *Amer J Geriatr Psychiatry, 4*, 197–207.

Tang NKY, Crane C. (2006). Suicidality in chronic pain: A review of the prevalence, risk factors and psychological links. *Psychol Med, 36*, 575–586.

Tao H, Guo S, Ge T, et al. (2013). Depression uncouples brain hate circuit. *Molec Psych, 18*, 101–111.

Tauber Y. (1998). *In the other chair: Holocaust survivors and the second generation as the therapists and clients.* Jerusalem, Israel: Gefen Publishing House.

Tavernise S. (2013, February 13). To reduce suicide rates, new focus turns to guns. Retrieved February 17, 2013, from *www.nytimes. com/2013/02/14/us/to-lower-suicide-rates-new-focus-turns-to-guns. html?pagewanted=all&_r=0.*

Taylor WD. (2014). Depession in the elderly. *N Engl J Med, 371*, 1228–1236.

Taylor CB, Youngblood ME, Cattellier D, et al. (2005). Effects of antidepressant medication on morbidity and mortality in depressed patients after myocardial infarction. *Arch Gen Psychiatry, 62*, 792–798.

Tess AV, Smetana GW. (2009). Medical evaluation of patients undergoing electroconvulsive therapy. *N Engl J Med, 360*, 1437–1444.

Tew JD, Mulsant BH, Houck PR, et al. (2006). Impact of prior inadequate treatment exposure on response to antidepressant treatment in late life. *Am J Geriatr Psychiatry, 14*(11), 957–965.

Thapa P, Gideon P, Cost T, et al. (1998). Antidepressants and the risk of falls among nursing home residents. *N Engl J Med, 339*, 321–237.

Thase ME, Macfadden W, Weisler RH, et al. (2006). Efficacy of quetiapine monotherapy in bipolar I and II depression: A double-blind, placebo-controlled study (the BOLDER II Study). *J Clin Psychopharm, 26*, 600–609.

Thompson LW, Gallager D, Breckenridge JS. (1987). Comparative effectiveness of psychotherapies for depressed elders. *J Consult Clin Psychol, 55*, 385–390.

Thompson LW, Gantz, F, Florsheim M, et al. (1991). Cognitive-behavioral therapy for affective disorders in the elderly. In WA Myers (Ed.), *New techniques in the psychotherapy of older patients* (pp. 3–19). Washington, DC: American Psychiatric Press.

Thompson LW, Coon DW, Gallagher-Thompson D. (2001). Comparison of desipramine and cognitive/behavioral therapy in the treatment of elderly outpatients with mild-to-moderate depression. *Am J Geriatr Psychiatry, 9*(3), 225–240.

Torpy JM, Burke AE, Glass RM. (2009). Coronary heart disease risk factors. *JAMA, 302*(21), 2388.

Toseland RW, Labrecque MS, Gooegel ST, et al. (1992). An evaluation of a group program for spouses of frail elderly veterans. *Gerontologist, 32*, 382–390.

Trejo JL, Carro E, Torres-Aleman I. (1996). Circulating insulin-like growth factor mediates exercise-induced increases in the number of new neurons in eh adult hippocampus. *J Neuroscience, 30,* 257–270.

Trivedi MH, Fava M, Wisniewski SR, et al. (2006a). Medication augmentation after the failure of SSRIs for depression. *N Engl J Med, 354,* 1243–1252.

Trivedi MH, Rush AJ, Wisniewski SR, et al. (2006b). Evaluation of outcomes with citalopram for depression using measurement-based care in STAR*D: Implications for clinical practice. *Am J Psychiatry, 163,* 28–40.

Turner A, Murphy BM, Higgins RO, et al. (2014). An integrated secondary prevention group programme reduces depression in cardiac patients. *Eur J Prev Cardiol, 21*(2), 153–162.

UK ECT Review Group. (2003). Efficacy and safety of electroconvulsive therapy in depressive disorders: A systematic review and meta-analysis. *Lancet, 361,* 799–808.

Umpierre D, Ribeiro PAB, Kramer CK, et al. (2011). Physical activity advice only or structured exercise training and association with HbA1c levels in type 2 diabetes: A systematic review and meta-analysis. *JAMA, 305,* 1790–1799.

Unützer J, IMPACT Study Investigators. (1999). *IMPACT intervention manual.* Los Angeles: UCLA Neuropsychiatric Institute, Center for Health Services Research.

Unützer J, Katon W, Callahan CM, et al. (2002). Collaborative care management of late-life depression in the primary care setting: A randomized controlled trial. *JAMA, 288,* 2836–2845.

Unützer J, Park M. (2012). Older adults with severe, treatment-resistant depression. *JAMA, 308*(9), 909–918.

Unützer J, Tang L, Oishi S, et al. (2006). Reducing suicidal ideation in depressed older primary care patients. *J Am Geriatric Soc, 54,* 1550–1556.

U.S. Department of Health and Human Services. (1996). *Physical activity and public health: A report from the Surgeon General.* Atlanta: National Center for Chronic Disease Prevention and Health Promotion.

U.S. Department of Health and Human Services, Agency for Healthcare Research and Quality. *Staying Healthy through Education and Prevention (STEP) implementation guide.* (2011). AHRQ Publication No. 10(11)-0076-EF. Rockville, MD: Author.

U.S. Department of Health and Human Services, Office of the Surgeon General, and National Action Alliance for Suicide Prevention. (2012). *National strategy for suicide prevention: Goals and objectives for action.* Washington, DC: Author. Retrieved September 2012, from *www.surgeongeneral.gov/library/reports/national-strategy-suicide-prevention/index.html.*

U.S. Preventive Services Task Force. (2003). *Counseling to promote a healthy diet in adults.* Retrieved October 25, 2010, from *www.uspreventiveservicestaskforce.org/3rduspstf/diet/dietsum.htm.*

U.S. Public Health Service. (1999). *The Surgeon General's call to action to prevent suicide.* Rockville, MD: U.S. Department of Health and Human Services.

U.S. Public Health Service. (2001). *National strategy for suicide prevention:*

Goals and objectives for action. Rockville, MD: U.S. Department of Health and Human Services.

van der Lee J, Bakker TJ, Duivenvoorden HJ, et al. (2014). Multivariate models of subjective caregiver burden in dementia: A systematic review. *Ageing Res Rev, 15,* 76–93.

van't Veer-Tazelaar N, van Marwijk H, van Oppen P, et al. (2006). Prevention of anxiety and depression in the age group of 75 years and over: A randomized controlled trial testing the feasibility and effectiveness of a generic stepped care programme among elderly community residents at high risk of developing anxiety and depression versus usual care. *BMC Public Health, 6,* 186.

Vasic N, Walter H, Höse A, et al. (2008). Gray matter reduction associated with psychopathology and cognitive dysfunction in unipolar depression: A voxel-based morphometry study. *J Affect Disord, 109,* 107–116.

Verghese J, Lipton RB, Katz MJ, et al. (2008). Leisure activities and the risk of dementia in the elderly. *N Engl J Med, 348,* 2508–2516.

Vickrey BG, Mittman BS, Connor KI, et al. (2008). The effect of a disease management intervention on quality and outcomes of dementia care: A randomized controlled trial. *Ann Intern Med, 145,* 713–726.

Waern M. (2003). Alcohol dependence and misuse in elderly suicides. *Alcohol Alcohol, 38,* 249–254.

Walker JG, Hansen CH, Hodges L, et al. (2010a). Screening for suicidality in cancer patients using item 9 of the nine-item patient health questionnaire: Does the item score predict who requires further assessment? *Gen Hosp Psychiatry, 32*(2), 218–220.

Walker JG, Mackinnon AJ, Batterham P, et al. (2010b). Mental health literacy, folic acid and vitamin B12, and physical activity for the prevention of depression in older adults: Randomized controlled trial. *Br J Psychiatry, 197*(1), 45–54.

Warner CH, Appenzeller GN, Parker JR, et al. (2011). Effectiveness of mental health screening and coordination of in-theater care prior to deployment to Iraq: A cohort study. *Am J Psychiatry, 168*(4), 378–385.

Webb RT, Kontopantelis E, Doran T, et al. (2012). Suicide risk in primary care patients with major physical diseases. A case-control study. *Arch Gen Psychiatry, 69*(3), 256–264.

Wei W, Sambamoorthi U, Olfson M, et al. (2005). Use of psychotherapy for depression in older adults. *Am J Psychiatry, 162,* 711–717.

Weintraub D, Rosenberg PB, Drye LT, et al. (2010). Sertraline for the treatment of depression in Alzheimer disease: Week-24 outcomes. *Am J Geriatr Psychiatry, 18*(4), 332–340.

Welle S. (1998) Resistance training in older persons. *Clinical Geriatrics, 6,* 48–59.

Wenzel A, Beck A, Brown GK. (2008). Cognitive therapy for suicidal older patients. In *Cognitive therapy for suicidal patients: Scientific and clinical applications* (pp. 263–282). Washington, DC: American Psychological Association.

Wethington E, Kessler RC. (1986). Perceived support, received support, and adjustment to stressful life events. *J Health Soc Behav, 27*, 78–89.

While D, Bickley H, Roscoe A, et al. (2012). Implementation of mental health service recommendations in England and Wales and suicide rates, 1997–2006: A cross-sectional and before-and-after observational study. *Lancet, 379*(9820), 1005–1012.

Whiteford HA, Degenhardt L, Rehm J, et al. (2013). Global burden of disease attributable to mental and substance use disorders: Findings from the Global Burden of Disease Study 2010. *Lancet, 382*, 1575–1586.

Whitlock EP, Orleans CT, Pender N, et al. (2002). Evaluating primary care behavioral counseling interventions: An evidence-based approach. *Am J Prev Med, 22*(4), 267–284.

Whitlock EP, Polen MR, Green CA, et al. (2004). Behavioral counseling interventions in primary care to reduce risky/harmful alcohol use by adults: A summary of the evidence for the U.S. Preventive Services Task Force. *Ann Intern Med, 140*(7), 557–568.

Whitney NP, Eidem TM, Peng H, et al. (2009). Inflammation mediates varying effects in neurogenesis: Relevance to the pathogenesis of brain injury and neurodegenerative disorders. *J Neurochem, 108*(6), 1343–1359.

Whooley MA. (2012). Diagnosis and treatment of depression in adults with comorbid medical conditions. *JAMA, 307*(17), 1848–1857.

Whyte EM, Rovner B. (2006). Depression in late life: Shifting the paradigm from treatment to prevention. *Int J Geriatr Psychiatry, 21*(8), 746–751.

Wilson KC, Mottram PG, Vassilas CA. (2008). Psychotherapeutic treatments for older depressed people. *Cochrane Database Syst Rev,* Jan 23;1:CD004853.

Windle G, Markland DA, Woods RT. (2008). Examination of a theoretical model of psychological resilience in older age. *Aging Ment Health, 12*(3), 285–292

Wisner KL, Perel JM, Peindl KS, et al. (2004). Prevention of postpartum depression: A pilot randomized clinical trial. *Am J Psychiatry, 161*, 1290–1292.

Woltman E, Grogan-Kaylor A, Perron B, et al. (2012). Comparative effectiveness of collaborative chronic care models for mental health conditions across primary, specialty, and behavioral health care settings: Systematic review and meta-analysis. *Am J Psychiatry, 169*(8), 790–804.

World Health Organization. (2008). *The global burden of disease: 2004 update.* Geneva, Switzerland: Author.

Wouts L, Oude Voshaar RC, Bremmer MA, et al. (2008). Cardiac disease, depressive symptoms, and incident stroke in an elderly population. *Arch Gen Psychiatry, 65*(5), 596–602.

Yan JH. (1999). Tai chi practice reduces movement force variability for seniors. *J Gerontol A Biol Sci Med Sci, 54*, M629–M634.

Yasavage JA, Karasu TB. (1982) Psychotherapy with elderly patients. *Am J Psychother, 36*, 41–55.

Yehuda R, Kahana B, Southwick SM, et al. (1995). Impact of cumulative lifetime trauma and recent stress on current post traumatic stress disorder symptoms in Holocaust survivors. *Am J Psychiatry, 152*(12), 1815–1818.

Zajecka J, Tracy KA, Mitchell S. (1997). Discontinuation symptoms after treatment with serotonin reuptake inhibitors: a literature review. *J Clin Psychiatry, 58*(7), 291–297.

Zanjani F, Mavandadi S, TenHave T, et al. (2008). Longitudinal course of substance treatment benefits in older male veteran at-risk drinkers. *J Gerontol A Biol Sci Med Sci, 63*, 98–106.

Zarit SH, Orr NK, Zarit JM. (1985). *The hidden victims of Alzheimer's disease.* New York: New York University Press.

Zarit SH, Reever KW, Bach-Peterson J. (1980). Relatives of impaired elderly: Correlates of feelings of burden. *Gerontologist, 20,* 649–655.

Zarit SH, Whitlach CJ. (1992). Institutional placement: Phases of the transition. *Gerontologist, 32,* 665–672.

Zarit SH, Zarit JM. (2006). *Mental disorders in older adults.* New York: Guilford Press.

Zisook S, Shuchter SR, Sledge P. (1994). Diagnostic and treatment considerations in depression associated with late-life bereavement. In LS Schneider, CF Reynolds III, BD Lebowitz, et al. (Eds.), *Diagnosis and treatment of depression in late life* (pp. 419–430). Washington DC: American Psychiatric Press.

Index

The letter *f* following a page number indicates figure; the letter *t* indicates table.

227